Health Informatics

Stephen Goundrey-Smith

Information Technology in Pharmacy

An Integrated Approach

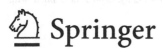 Springer

Stephen Goundrey-Smith, MSc.
Cert Clin Pharm, MRPharmS
SGS Pharma Solutions
Chedworth, Gloucestershire
UK

ISBN 978-1-4471-5837-0   ISBN 978-1-4471-2780-2 (eBook)
DOI 10.1007/978-1-4471-2780-2
Springer London Heidelberg New York Dordrecht

Printed on acid-free paper

Springer is part of Springer Science+Business Media (www.springer.com)

Preface

The purpose of this book is to provide a general introduction to pharmacy information technology at the current time, to discuss issues surrounding the adoption of technology and to discuss how technologies may be utilised by the pharmacy profession to exercise new professional roles and achieve new professional aspirations.

This has been a major project for me as a pharmacist, a health informatician and as a writer, and I would like to thank those whose assistance and support has been invaluable in the production of this book.

I am grateful to those who were of assistance with certain sections of the book.

- Hillary Judd and colleagues from First Databank Europe Ltd., for their input in the area of data support for electronic prescribing
- Joan Povey from JAC Computer Services Ltd., for providing screen views of the JAC electronic prescribing medicines administration module
- Garry McCrea, from the pharmacy department, Gloucestershire Hospitals NHS Trust, for photos of the Gloucester Royal Hospital pharmacy robot
- Dan Mandeman from the pharmacy department, Guys and St Thomas's NHS Trust, for photos of electronic ward cabinets at St Thomas's Hospital
- Donald MacIver, Manager of Cox and Robinson Pharmacy Ltd., Horsefair, Banbury, for photos and information on automated methadone dispensing

I am especially indebted, however, to those people with whom I have worked most closely on the electronic prescribing and pharmacy IT agendas over the past 10 years. In a sense, my expertise reflects theirs. They are (in no particular order):

- Former colleagues and associates from iSOFT – George Brown, Tom Bolitho, Clive Spindley, Tim Botten, Sue Braithwaite, Julie Randall and Raghu Kumar
- Heidi Wright from the Royal Pharmaceutical Society and Lindsay McClure from the Pharmaceutical Services Negotiating Committee
- Fellow members for the Guild of Healthcare Pharmacists/United Kingdom Clinical Pharmacy Association (UKCPA) IT Interest Group Committee

I would also like to thank:

- Alix Sibbald for his work on illustrations and diagrams
- Grant Weston and colleagues at Springer Verlag for their editorial support

Above all, I am grateful to my family – Sally, Edward, Archie, Sam and Emily – and friends in Chedworth for their support.

Chedworth, Gloucestershire, UK   Stephen Goundrey-Smith

Contents

1 IT Enabling Pharmacy Practice 1
Introduction. 1
IT in Pharmacy – Purpose and Scope. 2
The Profession of Pharmacy – Past, Present and Future 4
The Development of Clinical Pharmacy 6
The Development of Information Technology in Healthcare. 7
The Benefits of IT in Healthcare 9
The Quest for Intraoperability 9
Coding of Medicines Concepts 11
Medicine Item Codes. 15
Electronic Information Sources for Pharmacy and Therapeutics. .. 15
Electronic Drug Databases 18
Information Technology to Support the Medicines Use Process ... 20
Information Technology to Support Clinical Pharmacy 21
IT and the Interface Between Pharmacy and the
Pharmaceutical Industry 22
Clinical Safety. 23
Pharmacy IT as a Sociotechnical Innovation 24
Conclusion. 25
References. 26

2 Electronic Patient Records 27
Introduction. 27
Development of Electronic Patient Records 28
Legal and Professional Framework for EHRs 29
    Confidentiality. 29
    Consent. 30
    Liability. 30
Information Governance and Data Sharing 31
    UK Health Records Standards Initiatives 32
EHRs – Principles of Design and Use 34
    What Is an EHR? 34
    Systems Used for EPRs 34

Creation of EPRs 35
Access to EHR Systems by Pharmacy Professionals 36
Liability for Record Use............................... 37
Subject Access to EHRs............................... 38
Viewing the EHR 39
Sharing of Data 39
Use of Data for Purposes Other Than That for Which It Was
Collected.. 40
Business Continuity................................... 40
Archiving and Destruction of Records.................. 41
Electronic Health Record Initiatives 41
Benefits of EHRs 45
Clinical Pathways and Content 47
Optimisation of EPRs for Pharmaceutical Care.............. 48
Applications of EPRs for Pharmacists...................... 49
The Content of a Pharmaceutical Care Record 50
Medicines Reviews 51
Medicines Reconciliation 52
Shared Care 53
Long Term Condition Management 53
Homecare Supply 54
Appliances 54
Patient Group Direction (PGD) Supply 55
Public Health and Screening 55
Home Visits 55
Conclusions 56
References.. 56

3 **Electronic Prescribing and Medicines
   Administration in Hospitals** 59
   Introduction.. 59
   Benefits of Electronic Prescribing 60
   Reduction in Medication Error Rates with EP Systems 61
   Effect of EP Systems on Medication Error Rates in Paediatrics ... 66
   Role of Barcodes in EP Systems 67
   Increases in Medication Errors due to the Introduction
   of EP Systems 69
   Reduction of Medication Errors due to the Availability
   of Electronic Decision Support Tools at the Point
   of Prescribing 71
   Problems with Evaluating Risk Reduction
   Aspects of EP Systems 76
   Workflow Management for Clinical Users of EP Systems 78
   Discharge Process Efficiency................................ 82
   Facilitation of a Seamless Pharmaceutical Supply Chain 83

Reduced Use of Paper and Consumables 85
Clinical System Intraoperability 85
Improvement in Hospital Business Processes due to Electronic
Dissemination of Prescriptions 86
Security of Prescriptions and Prescribing Information 88
Quality of Care Benefits 88
Conclusion 89
References 90

4 **Pharmacy Automation** 95
History and Development of Dispensary Technology 96
Pharmacy Robot Design and Operation 97
Adoption of Pharmacy Automation in the UK 98
Drivers for Use of Automation in Pharmacy 100
Benefits of Pharmacy Robots 102
Evaluating the Benefits of Pharmacy Robots 105
Electronic Ward Cabinets 106
Benefits of Electronic Ward Cabinets 109
Implementation Issues with Electronic Ward Cabinets 110
Remote Dispensing Systems 112
Specialist Dispensing Systems 114
Conclusions 117
References 117

5 **Electronic Medicines Management in Primary Care** 121
The Development of Systems for Medicines Management
in Primary Care 121
Clinical Coding for GP Systems 124
Data Quality in GP Systems 126
GP System Functionality 126
    Identifying Patients and Registration 127
    Problem and Episode Recording 127
    Recording of Allergies 128
    Prescribing, Medication Records and Prescribing
    Decision Support Systems (DSS) 129
    Items of Service 131
    Pathology Tests 131
    Document Management 132
    GP to GP Transfer 133
    Data Migration 134
GP System Safety and Usability 134
Electronic Transfer of Prescriptions (ETP) 135
    Benefits of eTP 136
    eTP Functionality Issues 138
    Problems with eTP 142

Supplementary Clinical Information 142
Professional Checking.............................. 143
Substitution 143
Labelling of Prescriptions.......................... 144
Accuracy Checking 144
Owings and Out of Stock Items...................... 144
Dispense Notification 144
Submission of Reimbursement Endorsement Messages 145
Cancellation of Electronic Prescriptions 145
Electronic Repeat Dispensing........................ 145
Data Structure and Product Selection 146
Business Continuity................................ 146
Adoption of ETP.................................. 146
Prescribing Management Software.......................... 147
Conclusion.. 148
References.. 148

6   **Pharmacy Management Systems** 151
Introduction... 151
History and Development of Pharmacy Systems............. 151
Pharmacy System Requirements and Use.................. 152
Pharmacy System Architecture......................... 154
Community Pharmacy System Functions 155
Hospital Pharmacy System Functions 157
Stock Control Methodologies in Hospitals 158
Pharmacy System Interfaces 160
Reporting.. 161
Availability of Clinical and Medicines Information Through
Pharmacy Systems 162
System Functions 163
Benefits of Pharmacy Systems.......................... 164
Other Pharmacy Departmental IT Applications 166
Extension of EP Functions from Pharmacy Systems 168
Fridge Temperature Monitoring Software.................. 169
Integrated Community Pharmacy Systems 170
Systems to Support Clinical and Enhanced Services
in Community Pharmacy............................... 170
Conclusion... 171
References... 171

7   **Barcodes and Logistics**.................................... 175
Introduction... 175
Current Pharmaceutical Distribution Processes.............. 176
Development of Barcodes and Optical Technology............ 178
Radio Frequency Identification (RFID) 179

The Regulatory Framework for Supply Chain Harmonisation   179
Rationale for Barcode Symbology Harmonisation   181
Benefits of Barcode and Optical Technology in Pharmacy
and Medicines Management.................................   182
    Patient Safety...   182
    Security of the Supply Chain   184
    Tracking of Supply Chain Efficiency......................   184
    Intraoperability   185
    E-Commerce in Pharmacy..............................   185
    Reduction of Dispensing Errors   186
    Electronic Medicines Administration.....................   187
    Pharmacy Workflow Tracking   189
Conclusion..   191
References..   191

8 Future Prospects in Pharmacy IT...........................   193
Towards Integrated IT Systems in Pharmacy Practice...........   193
Smart Pumps...   195
Oncology Systems..   196
Challenges of Device Integration...........................   196
Smart Packaging...   197
Telecare and Pharmacy   201
Clinical Homecare   206
Methodology and Evaluation   207
Development of Professional Standards   208
Pharmacy Professional Engagement in IT Adoption.............   210
IT Education and Training..................................   212
Conclusion..   215
References..   215

Appendices   219

Index..   231

Chapter 1
IT Enabling Pharmacy Practice

Introduction

Over the last 30–40 years, information technology (IT) has revolutionised professional life for millions of people around the world. IT has reduced the need for bulk storage of paper records by organizations due to its capacity to store large amounts of digital data on hardware which is relatively small in size. Also, because IT systems can copy, process and disseminate data, and present data in different ways, computers have been able to automate tasks that were previously repetitive and labour-intensive, and carry them out in a fast and accurate way. For these reasons, the expansion of IT into the workplace – and indeed, the home – has completely changed working practices in many industries. IT has enabled economies of scale, improved efficiencies and enabled new ways of working that were hitherto impossible. The use of IT means that services can be provided to large populations, yet customised to each individual. Computers have had a major impact on many industry sectors including banking and finance, retail, the service industries – and healthcare.

In parallel with the rise of IT during the last 40 years, the role of the pharmacist – and the society in which pharmacists work – has changed considerably. Pharmacists are no longer principally compounders of medicines, as most medicines now are available in a suitably packaged form from manufacturers. However, pharmacists are still responsible for ensuring that the patient receives the correct medicine, ensuring that the patient understands why they should take their medicine, and helping the patient with taking the medicine and being concordant with therapy.

Modern medicines are becoming increasingly sophisticated in terms of their modes of action, so the information available about them is correspondingly more complex. Furthermore, the amount of medicines information available has increased exponentially, with information now available through a range of different providers. Traditionally, information on medicines was available in reference sources – pharmacopoeias and compendia – produced by specialist publishers and professional bodies, and also from the pharmaceutical industry. Today, however, medicines information is available from a plethora of sources on the internet.

S. Goundrey-Smith, *Information Technology in Pharmacy*,
DOI 10.1007/978-1-4471-2780-2_1, © Springer-Verlag London 2013

However, information provided over the internet will not be subject to the same quality processes and review mechanisms as information in the traditional medicine reference sources so, in some cases, this information may be biased or of questionable quality. A key issue is how the most appropriate information on medicines can be made available in the most readable form to the patient or healthcare professional at the point of care.

The increasing availability of medicines information direct to the patient, as with internet sources, means that information on medicines is no longer the sole preserve of the healthcare professional. There has also been an increase in the growth of consumerism in healthcare, with a corresponding reduction in paternalism on the part of the healthcare professional. People therefore see themselves as consumers of healthcare rather than patients. While, in fomer days, the doctor's advice was the final authority and was not questioned, now the patient will simply find a different clinician if they don't like the advice they receive. The concepts of the "empowered patient" and the healthcare professional as "a partner" with the patient in the healthcare process are now in common use among healthcare policy makers.

A combination of new medical technology and new information technology means that public health needs can now be identified and addressed in a way they could not in previous generations. And with the full understanding of public health issues, and the ability to address them, comes the ethical imperative to do so, with the corresponding pressures on health professional activity and healthcare provider budgets. Pressing public health issues, and their budgetary impact, especially in the deprived sections of the population, are huge drivers for the development of new professional roles in healthcare and the use of IT to enable these roles in both the United Kingdom and the United States. At the time of writing, the NHS in the UK is undergoing a far-reaching programme of reforms, which will have considerable impact on the efficiency of healthcare provision but, more subtly, on the relationship of different professional groups and how they might work together to optimise healthcare provision in the NHS. The UK NHS needs to realise huge cost savings in healthcare delivery – to the tune of approximately £20 bn – and many managers and clinicians recognise that these cost savings will only be realised through the use of IT systems in healthcare delivery, with the reduction of risk, increase in efficiencies, and the new ways of working that they enable.

IT in Pharmacy – Purpose and Scope

The book will describe some of the benefits and risks associated with the use of IT to support the provision of a pharmacy service, and some of the issues that pharmacy managers implementing these technologies face. The book will also explore the way in which current and emerging technologies might support new ways of working in pharmacy, to make the most of the pharmacist's skill set. IT applications that support the work of pharmacists in hospital and community pharmacy practice will be described and discussed, drawing on the author's experience and available research literature in the field. The emphasis will be on the holistic use of technologies to streamline and influence the prescribing and medicines use process, and so the book will look at IT systems that are not, or not solely, used by pharmacists, such as hospital electronic prescribing systems and the systems used in doctors' surgeries (GP systems).

Chapter 2 will look at the development of electronic health records, and the design, security and legal issues associated with them, and how the electronic health record can enable and optimise high quality pharmaceutical care. Chapter 3 will examine the benefits of hospital electronic prescribing (EP), the experiences of implementation and how it affects pharmacists. Chapter 4 discusses the various forms of automated dispensing that have been developed, including dispensary robots, ward cabinets, remote dispensing kiosks, and other forms of dispensing device. Chapter 5 will review the use of IT systems in the wider primary care arena, including general medical practitioner's systems, electronic transfer of prescriptions (eTP), and prescribing management systems and will describe the functions of these systems from a pharmacy perspective. Chapter 6 will examine the role of patient medication records in community pharmacy, and departmental pharmacy systems in hospital pharmacy, looking at their functions and their contribution to pharmacy management. Chapter 7 reviews the development of pharmacy logistics and how IT has impacted on this, particularly in the area of product and batch identification. Finally, Chap. 8 assesses potential future developments in IT to support pharmacy practice, together with the standards in education and professional development that will be required to capitalise on these.

The book will discuss the use of IT in pharmacy practice from an international perspective, looking at literature describing innovation and practice from different countries – most notably, the United States, UK, Europe and Australia.

The scope of the book does not extend to a full discussion of:

- The editorial and distribution processes for distributing reference sources on pharmacy and clinical medicine (eg formularies and monographs)
- The medicines information systems used purely to support the activities of the pharmaceutical industry
- Databases and systems used for the capture and storage of clinical trial data.

However, the discussion will touch on these areas to the extent to which they relate to the practice of pharmacy. The book describes pharmacy IT in general terms and is not intended to be a substitute for professional advice or consultancy in a specific practice setting.

As well as a discussion of the impact of technologies on pharmacy practice, this book will also discuss the issues surrounding the adoption and use of technology, the engagement of the pharmacy profession with technology, and the policy and standards that should underpin the use of technology by pharmacists. An exhaustive literature review of IT applications in pharmacy is beyond the scope of this book, although the book will refer to key research papers. Also, many of the IT applications and systems discussed are interrelated and there is an extent to which the division of the subject matter between the chapters is arbitrary.

In order to discuss the information requirements of the pharmacy profession and the role of IT in the working life of the pharmacist, it is necessary to review the history of the pharmacy profession [1], and the environments in which the profession operates.

The Profession of Pharmacy – Past, Present and Future

The profession of pharmacy emerged in the UK during the early nineteenth century, with a gradual distinction developing between apothecaries on the one hand, who were essentially medical practitioners, and chemists and druggists on the other, whose prime occupation was the preparation and supply of medicines. Some of these chemists and druggists were also apothecaries, others members of the pepperer's section of the Guild of Grocers and still others with no trade affiliation. However, following the Apothecaries Act of 1815, the activities of apothecaries were increasingly regulated, and there was a concern that, in emerging legislation, chemists and druggists who did not wish to become apothecaries would become subservient to the apothecaries. Consequently, a number of chemists and druggists decided to form a professional association to ensure that their interests were best served, and that they remained an independent group. The Pharmaceutical Society of Great Britain (Royal Pharmaceutical Society) was formed in 1841 for this purpose and soon established the legal basis for a register of pharmacists and a designation of pharmacist as a restricted title.

In Victorian times, in both the US and UK, pharmacists largely sold medicines rather than dispensed doctors' prescriptions (at that time pharmacists dispensed less than 10 % of prescriptions written by doctors in England and Wales). Furthermore, at this time, medicines were made of crude plant or animal extracts, and were of limited efficacy and often dubious quality. Many were produced in individual pharmacies according to a proprietary formula (secret recipe) of the pharmacist's choice. Consequently, during the early years of pharmacy, there was a large number of medicines available of variable formulae and quality and there was very little information available on these medicines, other than that compiled for advertising purposes.

In the UK, the 1911 National Insurance Bill signalled a change in how health services were provided, with a significant impact on the pharmacy profession. The National Insurance legislation established a national insurance scheme for those in employment, which provided free medical care – and medicines – for those contributing to the scheme. Previously, anyone consulting a medical practitioner would have paid a fee for the consultation, and a fee for any medicine prescribed at the consultation from the doctor's own dispensary. Under the national health insurance scheme, doctors would write prescriptions, which pharmacists would have the right to dispense. Because of the need for national health scheme reimbursement, the role of the doctor as prescriber and of the pharmacist as dispenser were separated. This had two effects. Firstly, it established a need for doctors and pharmacists to communicate about the dispensing of prescriptions. Secondly, there was a sharp increase in the percentage of doctors' prescriptions dispensed by pharmacists from around 10 % (as previously mentioned) to around 40 %. Income from prescription remuneration therefore became a major source of income for a pharmacy business. Local committees were established to process national health insurance scheme remuneration and a national Drug Tariff was introduced to standardise medicine prices and prescription payment processes.

These far-reaching changes in healthcare were further extended by the establishment of the National Health Service (NHS) in 1948, which aimed to provide free medical care (and medicines on prescription) to every citizen, not just those in employment.

The development of the welfare state in the UK, through the national insurance legislation of 1911 and the NHS Act of 1946, was the impetus for national standardisation of formulated medicines, and the availability of standard information on these medicines. As mentioned previously, in Victorian times, there had been a plethora of chemist's remedies of variable formula and quality available from pharmacies. However, following the introduction of the national insurance scheme in 1914, local reimbursement committees were urged not to pay for medicines with a "secret formula". This led to the development of a national formulary in 1929, which provided standard formulations for commonly-used unbranded medicines. This was the forerunner to the British National Formulary, one of the standard medicines reference sources in use today.

While the activities of the Pharmaceutical Society of Great Britain ensured that pharmacy began to emerge as a profession in the mid nineteenth century, pharmacists were still businessmen and a number of issues faced by pharmacists in the UK at that time related to their trade interests as much as to their professional standing. In 1880, a court action established a precedent that it was permissible for a corporate body to own multiple pharmacy premises. This was regularised in law in the 1908 Poisons and Pharmacy Act. This enabled the growth of multiple pharmacies in the UK, such as Boots, which had been established in 1877. There was therefore an increasing need for pharmacies to communicate with other branches of the same company, as well as with doctors and with their customers and patients.

Following the establishment of the NHS in 1948, the percentage of doctors prescriptions processed by the NHS rose to around 70 %, which is the figure at the current time. The formation of the NHS also therefore led to a reduction in the sales of proprietary medicines from pharmacies. However, while these trends might have been negative ones for pharmaceutical manufacturers, the industry was in a strong position with many new medicines being developed in the twentieth century "therapeutic revolution", and there was increased advertising activity for all medicines. A reaction to this was increased regulation of the medicine development and marketing process and the development of the Association of the British Pharmaceutical Industry Code of Practice on the advertising of medicines, introduced in 1958 [2] . These developments increased the amount of information on medicines available in the public domain, although many professionals have been concerned about how unbiased some of the information was. More recent developments on evidence-based medicine, such as the development of reviews such as the Cochrane Centre and National Prescribing Centre publications such as MeReC have attempted to ensure that balanced, evidence-based medicines evaluations are available to the health services.

Nevertheless, despite their "special" status, medicines are regarded in legal terms as ordinary items of commerce, as far as trading is concerned. In 1952, Boots the Chemists Ltd wanted to introduce self-service trade for medicines, which was already prevalent in the US, but the Pharmaceutical Society objected, arguing the medicines were not ordinary items of commerce, like other goods. This led to a High Court action in 1953, where the Pharmaceutical Society's argument was dismissed as protectionism, and which established that medicines could be traded in the same way as any other goods.

From the mid 1980s onwards, the policy direction of community pharmacy has been towards extended roles beyond dispensing. The 1986 Nuffield Report advocated extended roles for pharmacists, and the 1992 report, *Pharmaceutical Care: The Future of Community Pharmacy* made some important recommendations to support extended roles, such as:

• Pharmacists should maintain medication records for their patients
• Pharmacists should have consultation areas on their premises
• There should be a greater range of medicines available for sale over the counter to support pharmacy consultations and counter prescribing.

During the early twenty first century, these developments have largely been implemented in community (retail) pharmacy in England. Furthermore, a range of new services have been introduced in UK community (retail) pharmacy in the UK. These include the medicines use review (MUR), for reviewing medicines in the pharmacy, introduced under the 2005 English pharmacy contract, local enhanced services, which may include smoking cessation, needle exchange for intravenous drug users and minor ailments services, and, most recently, the new medicines service (NMS) for patients starting medicines for long term conditions. All of these have requirements for information management and storage, and processes have been developed to support pharmacists delivering these services.

The Development of Clinical Pharmacy

Critical to the explosion of information available on medicines, and the consequent need to systematise, store and retrieve that information has been the development of clinical pharmacy. An increase in the range of scientific techniques and processes available to the pharmaceutical industry, together with greater financial resources in the boom years after the Second World War led to the "therapeutic revolution" in the pharmaceutical industry with many innovative groups of medicines being developed, such as phenothiazine neuroleptics for schizophrenia, beta blockers for hypertension and angina, and H2 antagonists for gastric and duodenal ulcers. This led in turn to an increase in the amount of research literature and information available to prescribers. The greater number of medicines available, and the greater amount of information about them meant that hospitals had to adopt new procedures for the administration of medicines (the use of medicine charts (Kardexes) and drug trolleys) and that hospital pharmacists were increasingly required to provide advice on the use of medicines to doctors and nurses, rather than simply supply the medicines. In the UK, the 1953 Linstead Report recommended the involvement of hospital pharmacists in medical decision making and the 1958 Aitken Report stated that hospital pharmacists were responsible for safe and secure handling of medicines in the whole hospital, not just in the pharmacy department.

This led to the gradual development of clinical pharmacy, which may be defined simply as a pharmacy service at the patient's bedside, i.e. in a patient focussed manner. The US led the way with the development of clinical pharmacy services, such as near-patient pharmacy services, therapeutic drug monitoring and clinical specialism in pharmacy.

In the UK, the 1970 Noel Hall Report recommended a restructure of the hospital pharmacy service to make a better use of pharmacists' skills and recommended more research and development within hospital pharmacy. This led to the development of regional and district drug (medicines) information centres in the late 1970s and 1980s, providing a range of paper and electronic information sources on medicines, to support pharmacy practice and clinical pharmacy [3]. This has in turn led to routine post-graduate clinical pharmacy qualifications for hospital pharmacists, increased specialisation of pharmacists in different areas of medicine and therapeutics and the presence of clinical pharmacists, along with clinicians and nurses, on hospital wards rather than in the pharmacy department, during the 1990s. Ward-based, near-patient clinical pharmacists in UK hospitals today are often part of multidisciplinary teams and are supported by medicines management pharmacy technicians.

Information technology has already been developed to facilitate the processes of labelling, dispensing and supplying medicines, and to maintain patient medication records. Software applications are now available to deal with prescribing and medicines management beyond the dispensary, and many pharmacists are aware of, and are actively using, these applications. IT therefore has considerable potential to support pharmacists in future clinical roles, and to enable new approaches to pharmacy practice, as the twenty first century continues.

The Development of Information Technology in Healthcare

With the advent of solid state technology, where for the first time it was possible to build computers that were powerful enough to handle large volumes of data with optimal speed, but small enough to be of practical use in a working environment, organisations began to see the potential of computer-based systems to replace paper records of different sorts.

Within healthcare, the first major area of IT use in the 1970s was the collection and storage of patient data on a single computer to enable a healthcare provider to maintain electronic patient records, for administrative purposes. However, from around 1975 onwards, computers began to be used to automate manual, routine procedures and activities in US hospitals and clinics, and thus began to have a greater impact on clinical care. Assisted by the development of modern communications and networking technology, healthcare IT applications began to be integrated into larger, more sophisticated systems, which offered a range of functions to users within the organisation [4]. A pioneer of the move to bring computerised healthcare closer to patients was the John C. Lincoln Hospital in Phoenix, Arizona [5].

Consequently, over the last 30 years, systems have been developed to manage specific activities in hospital wards and departments. The most well-developed IT applications in secondary care have been pathology systems, for the management of test results, and pharmacy systems, for the labelling of dispensed items and for pharmacy stock control. Systems such as these were relatively straightforward to implement from a technical perspective, as they had their hub in one particular department of the hospital, and this department therefore had control over the implementation. However, the installation of a hospital departmental system represented a major change in working practice within a department, and had to be managed with care from a change management perspective.

In primary care, some clinicians actively embraced computer technology once personal computers were small enough for desktop use. However, the memory capacity of these early machines was limited and the coding of medicine concepts was necessary to enable large quantities of patient information to be stored in machine readable form. For this reason, Read codes were developed in the UK for coding medical terms on GP computer systems, and became pivotal in management of information in primary care. Coding systems also provided a common language so there was the potential for communication of information between systems in different practices, and production of comparable activity reports for a number of practices in a locality.

GP systems have been in use since the mid 1980s and offer a range of functions to support the working practices of GPs/primary care clinicians. These include storage of information on diagnoses and medical history, prescribing functions, provision of decision support functions for prescribing (interruptive DS for allergies, drug interactions etc, and availability of medicines reference information at the point of prescribing), pathology order management and items of service/billing and claim management.

Computers have been available to support prescribing in primary care for many years, and there is therefore considerable experience in this area, whereas the use of computers for prescribing in hospitals is at a much earlier stage of adoption. However, while GP systems were available to enable prescribing in medical practices back in the 1980s, their integration into the routine working practices of GPs has been much slower. By 1996, only one in four doctors were actually using their GP system in the course of a patient consultation [6].

The Benefits of IT in Healthcare

The main driver behind the adoption of IT in healthcare has been the various benefits that IT can provide for the organisation. Automated systems offer advantages over traditional paper-based systems in three main areas:

* Accuracy – automated systems can support the consistent use of medicine nomenclature, the accurate recording, display and transmission of prescription information, and the accurate display of clinical warnings as a result of a logical system of trigger points. Computers therefore are able to automate repetitive processes or monotonous processes which are prone to human error when carried out manually [7]. Thus automated systems are able to reduce clinical risk for the healthcare provider. An example of this is the use of IT to ensure accurate selection of medicines, where errors might arise from manual picking due to similar names, packs etc (see Fig. 1.1)
* Standardisation of data – automated systems allow patient data to be captured and stored according to standard formats and conventions. This facilitates the electronic transfer of patient data, and the production of comprehensive management reports. The production of management reports by hospitals and healthcare providers is an issue of great political significance in many healthcare economies where there is a need for governments and the public to be aware of healthcare issues and outcomes, and for healthcare providers to report on activity to payors and insurers. Furthermore, in standardising patient data, electronic systems therefore have the capacity for what has been described as "mass customisation" [7]. In healthcare terms, this means that, although the system handles large amounts of patient data, it is able to produce an individual care plan based on the specific personal requirements of each patient, thus supporting the personalisation of patient care in a consumerist society.
* Facilitating changes in working practices – automated systems have the capacity to process prescription information accurately and at scale, and are able to facilitate the display of that information in different contexts, according to system design and hardware availability. They are therefore able to make possible new ways of working for individuals and organisations. Because the system takes care of the routine recording, computational and transmission aspects of prescription information management, organisation processes may be restructured so that health professionals can engage with near-patient clinical activities, which require intuitive human qualities.

The Quest for Intraoperability

However, the issue facing all users of healthcare systems is that of their intraoperability. This has particularly been an issue in secondary care where a hospital has, historically, had a number of computer systems – a PAS, a pathology system, a pharmacy system, a radiology system – offering reliable functionality, but operating in parallel,

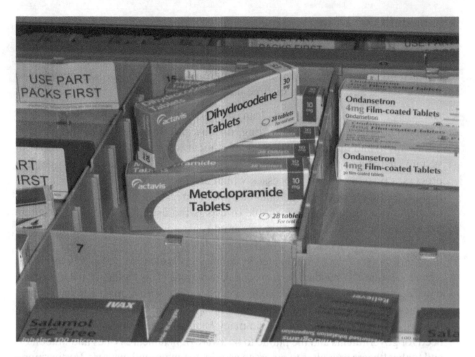

Fig. 1.1 Medication safety. Different medicines may have similar pack designs, which can cause dispensing errors; automated systems are able to avoid these errors

in a "silo" fashion, with no connectivity between them. This presents a number of problems – (a) duplication of effort in the design and configuration of functions that may be common to all systems (e.g. patient selection functions), (b) duplication of staff effort in data entry onto the systems, (c) introduction of risk due to all elements of a patient record not being visible to a user through a single system.

In many hospitals in the UK and US, a whole-hospital patient administration system (PAS) or hospital information system (HIS) has been installed, together with order communication systems, which deal with the messaging of orders in the broadest sense (e.g. radiology orders as well as pathology and pharmacy orders). However, these systems have traditionally relied on interface software to enable the central system to communicate with individual departmental systems. These interfaces are often complex to build and may themselves introduce data communication errors, and so require rigorous testing.

To enable systems to be truly intraoperable, standard data coding formats and terminologies are required so that healthcare applications will have a common database platform and can communicate in a common language. A number of standard coding systems, developed principally to record health events for public health purposes [8], can enable this as far as use of medicines is concerned. These include ICD 10 codes and DRG codes, Read codes and SNOMED CT codes, the HL7 terminology scheme and, specifically for medicines, the UK dm±d schema, which was developed as the basis of the UK NHS Connecting for Health applications.

Intraoperability has been a key aspiration of a number of regional and national healthcare IT systems, for example, the systems developed by US healthcare management organisations (HMOs) such as Kaiser Permanente, the UK NHS IT programmes, and schemes in Sweden [9] and Italy [10]. However, appropriate coding methodologies, and a willingness of all stakeholders to work towards an integrated system are essential to realise this goal. To understand current intraoperability issues with pharmacy IT and to appreciate the potential of future systems if data standards are incorporated, it would be helpful to have a discussion about the various coding schemas available for concepts associated with the prescribing and supply of medicines.

Coding of Medicines Concepts

If systems are to capture, store and transmit information about prescribing and medicines management, they require data schemas that will describe the concepts relevant to the prescribing and pharmacy domains. These would include:

1. Allergies
2. Medicine details (drug, strength, route etc)
3. Details of medicine administration duration
4. Current Diagnosis
5. Previous Medical History
6. Side-effects,

The discipline of health informatics has developed to analyse and systematise health and disease related information and, with time, a number of clinical coding systems have evolved to describe health and medicine concepts in a machine-readable manner [11]. Many of the coding systems have their historical origins in the need to classify and enumerate medical events for public health purposes. Many of these have relevance to EP systems and are discussed below.

The International Classification of Diseases (ICD) is a multiple axis disease classification schema which is published and administered by the World Health Organisation. It is now in its 10th revision (ICD 10), but the process is in place for developing the 11th revision [12], which will resolve issues such as usability on web-based systems and integration into electronic health records.

This schema has its origins in the work of William Farr, the first medical statistician for the General Register Office of England and Wales, in the mid-nineteenth century. He saw the need for a classification system for diseases to enable mortality statistics to be collected on an ongoing basis. Initially the schema was designed to record causes of death, but was subsequently developed to list diseases and disorders causing considerable morbidity. The classification continued to be used for the pragmatic purpose of collecting epidemiological data, and is currently used by WHO for making international comparisons of health statistics. The schema is therefore a practical classification, rather than a theoretical one, and it may require adjustments to allow finer levels of detail to be expressed in certain applications.

ICD 10 coding is often used as the coding system for diseases and diagnoses assigned to patients in electronic medical records, and would be the point of reference for medication management systems giving contraindication/precaution checking or drug-disease interaction checking, based on patient record information. ICD-10 codes are of particular concern in applications where there is a clear requirement for production of reports or statistical returns. An example of this would be oncology systems for the management of oncology and haematology clinics, where there is a major political need to report epidemiological data. In the UK, this is facilitated by the agreed National Cancer Data Set, which was established to eliminate reporting inconsistencies between different UK Cancer Registries [13]. The National Cancer Dataset is due to be replaced in 2012 by the Cancer Outcomes and Services Dataset (COSD), which will include the cancer registry dataset, and other site specific data items [14].

Diagnosis Related Groups (DRGs) were developed in the US by the Healthcare Finance Administration as a means of assigning a cost of treatment to a patient's diagnosis. They were developed to enable calculation of Medicaid reimbursement costs. DRGs are based upon ICD Clinical Modification (ICD-CM) codes in ICD 9 or ICD 10. Appropriate ICD codes are refined by placing them in diagnostic categories and then grouping them into subgroups that reflect consumption of resources, criteria for treatment, and potential complications. Thus patients are assigned a DRG from a relatively small number of DRG codes. DRGs are used routinely in the US and have been adapted in other countries where a reimbursement algorithm has been required. They are designed for hospital inpatients and do not provide a suitable means of assessing the costs of chronic disease care. Availability of a DRG designation for a patient, together with actual medicine cost data from an EP system may permit a variance analysis of projected costs and actual costs of inpatient treatment within the US context.

Read Codes (subsequently called Clinical Terms) were developed in the UK to enable clinicians (mainly in general practice) to code events in the electronic patient record, and thus enable statistical auditing of the patient care process in primary care. Read Codes have latterly been owned and administered by the UK government. Read Codes have changed considerably both in their terminology and in their structure during their lifespan. Version 1 of the Read Codes was a strictly hierarchical schema. In version 2, the structure was changed so that they more closely approximated ICD 9 disease codes and OCPS 4 procedure codes. Version 3 of the Read Codes was, in contrast with v1, a compositional schema, where each term could be augmented by qualifier terms.

While Read codes have been used extensively to code for diagnosis, problems and medicine prescribing in GP systems in the UK, they have not been used routinely in secondary care applications, largely because they were developed for primary care use. A key issue in the use of Read Codes has been the increasing potential for lack of concept control with combination terms, in the latter versions. However, many GP systems map prescribed medicines to their respective Read Codes, and Read Codes may therefore have a role in facilitating communication between primary care and secondary care systems in the UK.

The Systematised Nomenclature of Medicine (SNOMED) is administered by the College of American Pathologists, and was derived from classifications of tumour and pathology nomenclature used by the College. SNOMED is designed to be a comprehensive, computer processable terminology to support all medical concepts. SNOMED is in use in over 40 countries. Principally, it is a hierarchical, multiple-axis schema, but it also allows composition of complex terms from simple terms, so is partly compositional, and it has the facility of cross-referencing between terms in the schema. SNOMED International (SNOMED III) incorporates almost all ICD 9 terms, so reports can be generated in ICD 9 format.

In 1999, the College of American Pathologists and the UK National Health Service (NHS) announced their plan to converge SNOMED and Clinical Terms (Read Codes) v3 into a single terminology. The stated intention was to avoid duplication of effort and to create a universal, international terminology to support electronic patient records. The first version of the combined terminology – SNOMED Clinical Terms (SNOMED-CT) – was released in 2002, and was adopted as the standard terminology for England Connecting for Health healthcare applications [15]. Since 2007, SNOMED CT has been owned by the International Health Terminology Standards Development Organisation (IHTSDO). Third-party drug data suppliers have worked to map their datasets to international terminologies such as SNOMED-CT, in order to provide intraoperability with other systems in the area of more advanced decision support, for example contraindications, dose/indication checking and drug disease interactions.

An important area of data standardisation is the development of HL7 (Health Level 7), which is an XML based terminology [16], designed for the purpose of modelling healthcare processes, and producing a common terminology for all concepts in healthcare, to provide an industry standard for intraoperability across all healthcare applications. Many healthcare IT systems are marketed as "HL7 compliant" but it is worth bearing in mind that development of the message formats to enable extensive and comprehensive description of healthcare processes is an ongoing and gradual process. This is because (a) HL7 message formats are being designed to model all healthcare scenarios, not just those involving pharmacy and therapeutics, (b) there is a need for consistency in the consensus-forming process, and (c) major semantic assumptions need to be made and understood by the international HL7 community, at each stage of the HL7 design process in different domains. Recently, there have been initiatives to make closer links between SNOMED-CT concepts and HL7 message formats, in order to achieve greater semantic intraoperability in healthcare applications [17].

Specifically in the area of pharmaceuticals, the Dictionary of Medicines and Devices (dm ± d) has been developed to describe concepts associated with the use of specific medicines and devices for the diagnosis and treatment of patients [18]. The dm + d is integrated with SNOMED-CT and would enable applications dealing with medicines – such as hospital EP systems, and hospital and community pharmacy systems – to exchange information with a common terminology. The dm + d was developed as the medicines terminology for the English Connecting for Health programme. The first part of the dm + d work was the Primary Care Drug Dictionary,

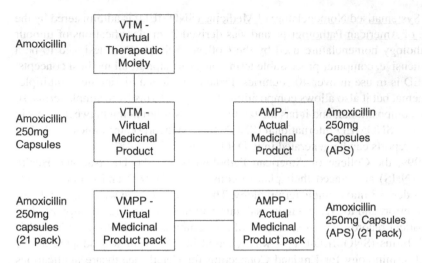

Fig. 1.2 dm+d structure

which was launched by the UK Prescription Pricing Authority in 2003. The first version of the full dm+d, for medicines used in primary care and secondary care, together with some prescribable devices, was released in 2004. Although the England NHS Connecting for Health programme is being dismantled, dm+d will become the standard for medicines terminology in the UK NHS, and will contribute to the intraoperability of systems in the NHS.

In order to support all aspects of the prescribing, supply and administration of medicines, the dm+d is structured into a number of related concepts, shown below (Fig. 1.2):

The dm+d data structure enables systems to differentiate at the data level between the concepts of medicine prescribing, administration and supply, which is important to provide rich functionality at each stage in the medicines management process.

Use of the dm+d will have a number of important benefits for patient care:

1. It will enable users to identify prescribed medicines clearly and unambiguously on systems, which will have a positive impact on patient safety.
2. It will also provide a common platform for analysis of prescribing data in both primary and secondary care in the UK, something that cannot be done at present. This will have important implications for commissioning and care management.
3. Comprehensive linkage of dm+d codes with GTIN codes (formerly EAN codes) will enable widespread and reliable use of automation in hospitals and healthcare provider organizations, in conjunction with hospital and health provider EP systems.
4. Use of dm+d will enable a common terminology to be developed to describe dosage instructions for medicines (dose syntax), which will enable greater intraoperability between prescribing and dispensing systems (GP systems and hospital EP systems, and pharmacy systems)

Medicine Item Codes

The ability to identify individual medicine formulations and packs clearly and without ambiguity is a pre-requisite for using IT to manage the automated supply and electronic administration of medicines, as well as to track the movement of medicines through the supply chain from manufacturer to patient. The use of machine-readable coding systems to describe medicine packs is therefore an important aspect of using IT to support the medicines supply process.

The EAN code is the international numerical code that supports a product barcode. EAN stands for European Article Number, but the coding system used is now correctly referred to as the GTIN code. Some years ago, the UK NHS Purchasing and Supply Agency (PASA) (now the Commercial Medicines Unit of the Department of Health) recommended that, where possible, all pharmaceutical products used in the UK NHS should be assigned an EAN code. Manufacturers have to apply for a manufacturer's code, so that their EANs don't clash with those of other manufacturers, and would then apply for codes for their products [19]. The EAN and barcode is essential if the product is going to be used in any automated dispensing system or pharmacy robot.

The PIP (Pharmaceutical/Pharmacist Interface Product) code is a coding system specifically to support the pharmaceutical wholesaler supply chain in the UK. It is of importance when pharmaceutical products are distributed via wholesalers. The PIP code system is owned by CMP Medica Ltd, the owners of Chemist & Druggist, and is linked in with the C&D Price List. There is a significant minority of pharmaceutical products in the UK which do not have PIP codes, and there have been some problems in recent years with accessioning and expansion with the PIP code system. PIP codes are, however, not machine-readable like the EAN code, and are not used by IT systems for medicines management.

Electronic Information Sources for Pharmacy and Therapeutics

Also foundational for an understanding of IT systems that support pharmacy professional activity is an understanding the types of medicines information that a prescriber or pharmacist might need to know, and the established reference sources that are available for prescribers and clinical professionals. Much of this will be familiar to practicing pharmacists, but is discussed here for the benefit of informatics professionals and students of all disciplines.

Historically, sources of drug information have consisted of

(a) medical and pharmaceutical primary literature from hardcopy journal publications
(b) secondary literature, such as recognised pharmaceutical compendia and reference books

The primary literature consists of clinical trial reports, reviews of specific therapeutic issues, case studies and anecdotal reports. The secondary literature consists of drug information compiled from primary sources. This might include recognised reference books, addressing specific clinical issues, such as Stockley's "Drug Interactions", or Briggs' "Drugs In Pregnancy". The secondary literature also comprises of recognised pharmaceutical compendia. A compendium is a book, with a section or monograph, on each listed medicinal product or drug substance. Some of the compendia provide standards for manufacturing and quality control purposes (for example, the British Pharmacopeia and the European Pharmacopeia) and are of little value for prescribers and clinical professionals. Others contain more evaluated clinical information (for example, the Martindale Extra Pharmacopeia), or provide treatment guidelines for rapid reference (for example, the British National Formulary (BNF), Physicians Desk Reference (PDR) or the Monthly Index of Medical Specialities (MIMS)).

Since automated systems have allowed substantial indexed databases to be compiled, stored and retrieved electronically, medical publishers and medical information providers have sought to provide their information sources to end-users in an electronic format. Initially, in the 1970s and 1980s, these electronic products were abstract database services such as the US National Library of Health Medline database, or the Exerpta Medica EMBASE, provided by hosted data services accessed by modem connection – for example, DataStar and Dialog – which enabled remote users to search proprietary databases and information sources. In the last decade or so, with the growth of the internet, many of these database services have become available via web browsers, which have made access far more straightforward and has simplified searching techniques, enabling a higher degree of end-user access.

Also, with the introduction of optical disk technology over the last 20 years, many of the biomedical databases have been "packaged" and sold as CD-ROM products for single and multi-user use, to enable fast and secure local searching. Many of the pharmaceutical compendia – for example, the British National Formulary or the Martindale Extra Pharmacopeia – are also now available in electronic format, on CD-ROM for single-user or network access.

It should be noted that there are many different databases of medicine-related information that are produced by commercial vendors, professional societies and public bodies, in different countries. An increasing number of these reference sources have been designed specifically for internet use, which enables them to be linked with other systems, and to be accessed by patients and health service end users, rather than health professionals (Clinical Knowledge Summaries (CKS), Map of Medicine, patient.co.uk).

Examples of some of these are tabulated below (Table 1.1):

In addition to information about medicines produced and compiled by healthcare professional bodies, health providers and the publishing industry, a prime source of information on medicines is from the manufacturers of those medicines. A number of key documents on licensed medicines are made available by the pharmaceutical industry and regulatory agencies. These include:

1. The Summary of Product Characteristics (SmPC). This is the definitive document on a marketed medicine for use by healthcare professionals. It provides a full listing of available data on a medicine in medical terminology.

Table 1.1 Sources of electronic medical information

Database	Geographical emphasis	Speciality
MedLine	US/UK	Medical Research
EMBASE (Excerpta Medica)	Europe	Clinical Medicine
TOXBASE	UK	Drug Toxicity and Side Effects
PharmLine	UK	Clinical Use of Drugs/Pharmacy Practice Research
TICTAC	UK	Medicines Identification Database
IDIS (Iowa Drug Information Service)	US	Clinical medicine and medicines information
Clinical Knowledge Summaries (formerly Prodigy)	UK	Treatment guidelines
Map of Medicine	UK	Treatment pathways and guidelines
Patient.co.uk	UK	Patient information on medicines

2. Thе Patient Information Leaflet (PIL). This is the approved information on a medicine that is available to a patient. The PIL is usually written in plain English, with non technical language. The PIL is included in each medicine pack and, in countries where original pack dispensing is not universal, such as the UK, there is a legal and ethical requirement for the pharmacist to include a copy of the PIL in the dispensed pack.
3. The European Public Assessment Document (EPAD). This is the document produced by a pharmaceutical company, under the auspices of the European regulatory system, giving a summary of the information supporting the product license application for a medicine.

It is often thought that information provided by the pharmaceutical industry is inferior to that available from independently published sources. However, the required content of the standard medicines documents, the SmPC and the PIL, is now highly controlled and regulated, and therefore these documents form a reliable source of definitive information on a medicine. Furthermore, since the introduction of the structured SmPC format some years ago, much of the information available to health professionals from the pharmaceutical industry in the UK and Europe is presented in a structured way, which could be incorporated into electronic systems. The SmPCs and PILs for UK authorizations are available online in the Electronic Medicines Compendium (EMC).

The availability of medicines information in various electronic formats brings with it the opportunity of linking that information (mounted either on a local network, or on the internet) to electronic systems for prescribing and medicines management. Indeed, many EP systems have implemented controls to link passively to standard electronic medicines reference sources, in order that these reference sources may be used as explicit decision support tools, although there may be issues concerning licensing in a multi-user situation, or with performance if the reference source is mounted on a remote server. Moreover, medicines information reference sources encoded as XML are particularly suitable for access by EP systems. For example, there has been an initiative in the UK to produce PILs in XML format (X-PILs) to enable PILs to be easily adapted to different formats, to enable access by people who are blind or partially sighted [20].

Electronic Drug Databases

Although electronic versions of hard-copy medicines reference sources constitute high quality sources of medicines data, they are often not suitable for direct use as a data source within pharmacy and medicines management software applications for a number of reasons. Firstly, they were compiled for referential purposes, not to support data retrieval in automated systems. This is to say that they were designed for use by a human evaluator and do not have the detailed linkages to support information retrieval by an automated system. Secondly, the data are not always structured or defined in an appropriately granular manner for use in an electronic system to support complex prescribing. Thirdly, the data are often not linked with appropriate coding systems to allow interoperability with other systems and to support a variety of advanced functions.

For these reasons, many electronic prescribing and pharmacy systems use drug databases that are structured to support the functions of the system. The standard data items – drug name, form, strength, synonyms, possible routes, units of prescribing, administration and supply etc – are all incorporated into data tables within a standard database platform, such as MicroSoft SQL Server. The database tables are structured so as to provide appropriate granularity to permit a range of detailed functionalities (for example, complex prescribing and medicines administration) and are linked in such a way as to provide consistent retrieval of information on medicines and prescribing concepts by the EP system, together with the possibility of incorporating mappings to other drug coding systems (e.g. SNOMED CT, dm±d, Read 2).

Currently, the most prominent of third party data providers for the provision of drug data to EP and medicine management system suppliers are First Databank Inc and First Databank Europe Ltd, owned by the Hearst Corporation, and Multum, part of the Cerner Corporation. Other sources of drug data include the MicroMedex product range (Thomson Inc), although these products are designed more for use with stand-alone hand-held devices.

Historically, third party data suppliers for IT system have not provided referential medicines information to end users, although they have had the capacity to do so; this has been the preserve of the reference sources produced by the publishing sector. However, recently First Databank Europe Ltd has marketed the medicines referential information that supports its decision support functions in a web-based browser format for end-user use (FirstLight ®). With increasing data transfer and adaptability, and the need for large information providers to find new markets, this trend is likely to continue.

In the US, some authors have in the past questioned the quality of data from third party data suppliers [21]. However, as commercial organisations whose principal business is supplying medicines data, third party data suppliers review their quality maintenance systems on a continual basis, and are often looking to introduce more advanced functionality. It should be noted too that, in the US, the major centres of excellence for hospital EP systems have the resources and in-house expertise to produce institutional drug databases [21]. However, other smaller healthcare providers do not have the means to produce their own drug reference files and it could be argued that more widespread adoption of EP systems cannot take place without the adoption of third party data sources. Indeed, many of the hospitals in the UK with operational EP systems use data from First Databank Europe Ltd (Exeter) [22–24].

The drug data used to support any system with a prescribing or pharmacy application may be compiled in one of three ways.

(a) The drug database is built for the implementation, by personnel within the organisation implementing the system. This approach has been taken with certain general hospital clinical systems that have been adapted for the application of prescribing. However, the build process is time-consuming and laborious and it is highly unlikely that the dataset will have the internal consistency of a commercially produced system. Furthermore, the implementing site has the burden of maintaining the system to reflect new products, changes in dose etc, which may not be feasible depending on the scope of the system or the resources available to maintain the system.

(b) The drug database is adapted from a software vendor's reference database, or a database from another implementation. However, with system providers' in-house databases, there may not be a systematic validation process in place, and the quality of the maintenance process will depend on the expertise and management structures in place within the software provider organisation. Often, with databases built by software houses, where developers may be working both on the software code and the data tables, there may be the temptation to provide some data-related functionality via hard-coded software changes, and thus the boundary between the data and the software can become indistinct. Furthermore, if a database from one implementation is used to support a new implementation, it may introduce data that are inappropriate to a different healthcare setting, and errors in the database are perpetuated. Furthermore, if the database has been compiled by a healthcare provider, there may be legal issues surrounding the ownership of the data.

(c) The drug database is structured around, and the data imported from, a third party data supplier dataset. The use of a third party dataset has the advantage that it is more likely to be of a higher quality than a database built by a software vendor or healthcare provider. Third party drug data providers are commercial organisations whose business is to produce databases to support medicines management software, and will have considerable expertise – both clinical and information science – available to them. The dataset of a third party data supplier should be consistent and accurate, with established business processes in place for the compilation and validation of their data. Furthermore, some of these organisations will have external validation, according to quality standards such as ISO 9001. The use of a third party dataset removes the responsibility of maintenance from the software vendor, or the healthcare provider (although some data configuration by the software vendor may be required). Also, with a third party data supplier, the legal responsibility for the internal quality of the drug data lies with the data supplier. The major disadvantage with using a third party dataset is the cost of using the data. Typically, a third party data supplier will charge a software vendor for the basic cost of supplying the data, together with an additional charge based on the number and size of sites where the system using the data is in use. These costs are factored into the total contract between the software vendor and healthcare provider, but it still increases the total cost of the implementation. Furthermore, the process of implementing a third-party dataset into a system that has not previously been supported by one will constitute a major technical task, which may deter some system providers and their users from migrating to a third party data supplier.

Information Technology to Support the Medicines Use Process

Traditionally, the role of the pharmacist in healthcare has related to the preparation and supply of medicines. However, over the last 30 years, an increasing number of medicines have become available in original packs from pharmaceutical manufacturers, and the role of the pharmacist in hospital and community has moved away from being purely concerned with the extemporaneous preparation and supply of medicines. Pharmacists are experts in the actions, formulation and practical use of medicine and therefore have an important advisory role in the use of specific medicines in patient care, but also on the use of medicines in general, and the processes and activities in which medicines are used. Pharmacists have a major impact on medicines use processes in hospitals, both as specialists concentrating on safe and effective use of medicines in their clinical specialism and also as generalists looking at the use of medicines in the hospital as a whole. In both hospital and community pharmacy, pharmacists may also be involved with providing services for medicines review, management of long-term conditions and public health/screening services. A variety of computer applications have been developed to support the medicines use process, and to facilitate the pharmacist's extended role. Many of these applications draw upon the medicines information sources, electronic databases and coding systems and schemas described above to enable their functional features.

Such applications might include:

1. Electronic health records (within either GP or pharmacy systems), which enable the detailed recording of a patient's medication history, and provide decision support to the pharmacist when the record is accessed or further information entered

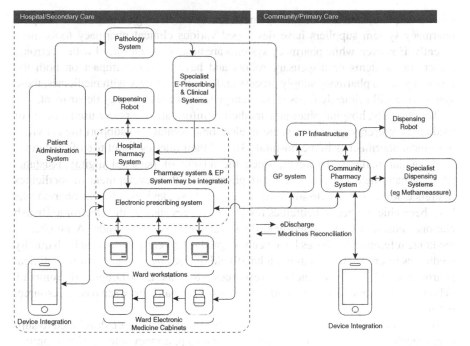

Fig. 1.3 An integrated IT system to support pharmacy practice

2. <u>Pharmacy system</u> functions for dispensing, labelling and stock control of medicines.
3. <u>Electronic prescribing</u>/ordering and medicines management.
4. <u>Pharmacy automation</u> to enable a seamless supply chain and facilitate medicines management on a hospital ward.
5. Hand held devices containing pharmacokinetics (drug metabolism) calculators or medicines information for referential use in clinical settings
6. <u>Pharmacy tracking</u> software, for workload management
7. <u>Pharmacy intervention logging</u> and reporting tools

Many of these applications are covered in greater detail in subsequent chapters. The diagram above indicates how these systems might interface with each other (Fig. 1.3).

The next section will provide some further detail on IT applications that support the practice of clinical pharmacy, primarily in hospitals.

Information Technology to Support Clinical Pharmacy

Departmental pharmacy systems in hospitals were developed primarily for the operational management of the pharmacy department and dealt primarily with processes such as dispensing and <u>labelling</u>, <u>stock control</u>, <u>ordering</u> and <u>ward stock inventories</u> (see Chap. 6). These systems were not originally designed to support clinical pharmacy

– i.e. near-patient medicines management activities, although many of the hospital pharmacy system suppliers have developed various clinical pharmacy tools more recently. However, while pharmacy systems are now often interfaced with electronic prescribing systems or dispensary robots and have a greater impact on both the efficiency of the pharmacy supply process and on patient safety with medicines, these systems are still primarily focused on management of the pharmacy department.

Traditionally, hospital pharmacy medicines information services used a range of medicines reference sources – some in electronic format – to support the activities of clinical pharmacists in the hospital [3], and their queries about use of medicines in particular patients. However, since the advent of personal digital assistants (PDAs), hand-held devices and smart phones and the development of medicines reference sources in electronic form to go on these devices, clinical pharmacists have been able to access medicines reference sources such as the electronic British National Formulary on a hand-held device at the patient's bedside. A number of medicine reference databases have been adapted specifically to provide high quality medicines reference information on hand-held devices by medical staff and clinical pharmacists [25]. These include resources such as Lexi-Drugs, Micromedex (Thomson Inc) and, more recently, the First Databank browser-based resource, FirstLight.

In addition to these a variety of stand-alone systems have been developed to support specific aspects of clinical pharmacy, such as pharmacy intervention monitoring, pharmacokinetics and therapy monitoring and patient information. These and other clinical pharmacy applications will be discussed in greater detail in Chap. 6 on pharmacy systems.

IT and the Interface Between Pharmacy and the Pharmaceutical Industry

In their early days, a number of major pharmaceutical manufacturers were founded and managed by pharmacists, and historically, the pharmacy profession has had a major role and influence within the pharmaceutical industry. However, in the more recent past, a growth in the number of life science graduates of other disciplines, together with the changing roles of pharmacists and differences in remuneration for pharmacists in industry compared with the other branches of pharmacy, have meant that there are fewer pharmacists in the pharmaceutical industry today. Furthermore, pharmacists in the NHS have always treated the pharmaceutical industry with caution and recent trends in the NHS towards evidence-based medicine and more rigorous Health Technology Assessments (HTAs) have accentuated this uneasy relationship. For all of these reasons, there is now a clear distinction between the pharmaceutical manufacturing industry as a seller of medicines, and pharmacy industry – wholesalers, buying groups, multiples and independent pharmacies – who are the buyers of medicines.

However, IT systems and machine-readable codes help to bridge the gap between pharmacy and the pharmaceutical industry to enable a seamless pharmaceutical supply chain, to provide appropriate information on medicines from the industry to pharmacy users, and to enable medicines to be available for prescription.

- The use of EAN UCC barcodes (EAN codes) enables products to be identified at any stage of the supply chain – by sorters on pharmaceutical company production lines, automated picking devices at wholesalers, pharmacy robots or electronic cabinets on wards or at clinic locations. Adoption of newer barcode conventions, which will enable storage of more data will enable batch numbers and expiry dates to be included in a machine-readable form and will facilitate product tracking and automated product recall.
- The internet can be used as a means for pharmaceutical companies to make proprietary product information available to patients and to healthcare professionals. With increased use of smart phones and hand-held devices, these information sources can be made available in an increasingly personal and portable manner. The challenge for the pharmaceutical industry will be for it to develop applications that do more than simply meet its marketing needs, but which provide a valuable service to healthcare professionals and patients. Such applications could also be used to deal with industry-wide issues such as adverse event reporting or monitoring medicine compliance.
- Pharmaceutical companies provide information on a new medicine (including EAN code, PIP code, pack details and price) for third party data suppliers such as First Databank, which is then used to supply GP and pharmacy system suppliers, or which may be submitted directly to system suppliers, in those cases where the system suppliers compile their own drug database. The data or system supplier ensures that a product file for the new medicine is included on their database – and this enables the medicine to be prescribed and dispensed in the health service. However, in order for the medicine to be prescribable locally, the new product information needs to be cascaded from the data supplier to the system supplier (if applicable) and then supplied to individual GP and pharmacy system installations in (usually) a monthly data update. However, problems can arise depending on (a) how data from a data supplier are implemented in a specific system, (b) how often updates are implemented by destination sites and (c) how destination site software is configured to display drug data.

Clinical Safety

As mentioned previously, one of the key benefits of automated systems in healthcare is their ability to reduce the risk of human error in work activities that are repetitive, require attention to complex detail or are inherently boring. For these reasons, IT systems have the potential to reduce errors associated with the prescribing, dispensing and administration of medicines.

However, it is known that risks associated with medicine and healthcare are often multifactorial and that having established processes and procedures in place within the organisation for staff to follow helps to mitigate this risk. Consequently, as well as the reactive testing of specific systems during the installation process, proactive clinical safety standards have an important role to play in the design and implementation of healthcare systems, including those involved with the medicines use process.

There is a distinction between clinical risk, and risk that is associated primarily with system usability. However, in reality, these two are interlinked, because poor system usability will lead to operator error which will introduce clinical risk.

In 2009, the UK NHS Information Standards Board issued guidance to establish software safety management regime in the health sector. These were comparable with safety standards in industries such as aviation or nuclear power, where safety and prevention of critical incidents has long been a concern. These safety standards, DSCN 14/2009 (for suppliers) and DSCN 18/2009 (or health organisations) require the proactive risk assessment and mitigation for IT systems used to support healthcare activities, but which are not medical devices. These standards would be applicable for all systems which might be used for direct patient care, such as GP systems, hospital EP systems and other specialist clinical systems.

Under these standards, health provider institutions in England are required to:

- Seek to procure systems which comply with DSCN 14/2009 (the supplier safety standard)
- Perform a risk assessment when rolling out a new system
- Ensure any risks identified are properly understood, investigated and mitigated by sensible controls (such as checks on migrated data or local testing to ensure the new system is correctly configured)
- Ensure that there is a clearly defined process for reporting safety issues to system suppliers.

Safety standards are also being developed for interfaced devices, such as glucose meters, which can automatically send data to electronic health records. These include IEC80001, introduced in 2011, which will require health providers to properly document and risk-assess systems and network components, which interface with medical devices.

Health professionals, including pharmacists, should have opportunities to influence organisational decisions, both in terms of IT systems and working policies and processes, which could have a systemic effect on clinical safety Some risks will be mitigated by technical solutions, either relating to the data, software or configuration, or by user guidance, or maybe a combination of both. For some risks that are dependent largely on human behaviour or professional 'best practice', the best mitigation may be user guidance, which users understand, and can see why it has been put in place.

Pharmacy IT as a Sociotechnical Innovation

Much is made of the capacity of IT systems to automate processes and therefore to (a) ensure that repetitive process are carried out fast and accurately, (b) provide consistency of process through standard coding and terminology, and (c) to enable new ways of working through process change. However, it must be remembered that the accurate operation of systems requires accurate input from human operators too. The stock phrase about human error with computers, "garbage in, garbage out" is apposite.

Systems have thus been described as a "sociotechnical innovation" [26] – meaning that they rely not just on computer hardware and technology, but the intuitive input of human beings, as part of the total environment in which they operate. With hospital electronic prescribing systems, it has been noted that the ability of systems to reduce medication errors relies not only on the operation of the software, but also the interaction of people with the software at the point of use. For this reason, system usability is important, and has been subject to considerable research using a variety of methods [27]. It is known from the experience with the Electronic Prescription Service (EPS) in England that end user systems can be compliant with the common assurance process (CAP) from a technical and functional perspective, but have problems with system usability when a person is put in front of the system.

One of the big debates in system design is whether systems should fit around, and automate, existing processes, or whether working processes should be reverse-engineered to fit an IT system. As a general rule, the former situation is preferable and makes introduction of IT easier. However, many systems are highly configurable and the possibility exists for systems to be configured to enable a new way of working, which would not have been possible without the ability of the system to automate and speed up monotonous and repetitive processes. Nevertheless, if a system is configured to support a new way of working, then proportionally more user training is required to ensure that the new working practice is safe and efficient.

Conclusion

The profession of pharmacy has traditionally been concerned with the preparation, dispensing and supply of medicines. However, during the last 30 years, due to the increasing complexity of modern medicines, the need to evaluate new medicines and wider changes in the health service, pharmaceutical industry and society in general, new professional roles have emerged for pharmacists. During this time, information technology has developed considerably and is able to support new roles and new ways of working for pharmacists. There is now the potential for IT systems to support the medicines use process and pharmacy professional activity in an integrated manner. However, an appropriate data, coding and classification infrastructure for medicine and pharmacy concepts is essential to underpin this. There is also a need for convergence between a range of systems that historically have been designed and developed separately, in order to deliver integrated medicines management services.

References

1. See Anderson S. Making medicines. London: Pharmaceutical Press; 2005. p. 77–94.
2. Prescription medicines code of practice authority. ABPI code of practice. 2012:6. www.pmcpa. org.uk/files/sitecontent/ABPI_Code_2012.pdf. Accessed August 2012.
3. Smith SJ, Bottle RT. Use of information sources by drug information pharmacists. Pharm J. 1994;253:499–501.
4. Burleson K. Review of computer applications in institutional pharmacy – 1975–1981. Am J Hosp Pharm. 1982;39:53–70.
5. Borggren L. Computers in pharmacy: improve efficiency and productivity. Comput Healthc. 1984;5(7):39–40.
6. Gillies A. Information and IT for primary care. Oxford: Radcliffe Press; 2000. p. 3.
7. Bates DW, Gawande AA. Improving safety with information technology. N Engl J Med. 2003;248:2526–34.
8. Goundrey-Smith SJ. Principles of electronic prescribing. London: Springer Science; 2008. p. 77–84.
9. Sjoborg B, Backstrom T, et al. Design and implementation of a point-of-care computerised system for drug therapy in Stockholm metropolitan health region – Bridging the gap between knowledge and practice. Int J Med Inform. 2007;76:497–506.
10. For example, the Umbrian regional healthcare system in Italy (see Barbarito F. Regional service card health and social care information system. Presented at opportunities in e-Health, London, 30 Nov 2006).
11. Coiera E. Guide to health informatics. 2nd ed. London: Arnold; 2003. p. 202–22.
12. Ustun TB. Presented at Australian Health & Welfare Institute meeting, Towards ICD 11 for Australia. University of Sydney. 2011. http://www.aihw.gov.au/TwoColumnWideLeft. aspx?pageid=10737419473. Accessed January 2012.
13. Pheby DF, Etherington DJ. Improving the comparability of cancer registry treatment data and proposals for a new national minimum dataset. J Public Health Med. 1994;16:331–40.
14. National Cancer Intelligence Network. Cancer outcomes and services dataset. 2011. http://www. ncin.org.uk/collecting_and_using_data/data_collection/ncds.aspx. Accessed January 2012.
15. NHS connecting for health electronic prescribing in hospitals: challenges and lessons learnt. 2009. p. 74. http://www.connectingforhealth.nhs.uk/systemsandservices/eprescribing. Accessed January 2012.
16. Kabachinski J. What is health level 7? Biomed Instrum Technol. 2006;40:375–9.
17. Ryan A, Eklund P, et al. Toward the intraoperability of HL7v3 and SNOMED CT: a case study modelling mobile clinical treatment. Med Info. 2007;12:626–30.
18. Frosdick P, Dalton C. What is the dm + d and what will it mean for you and pharmacy practice? Pharm J. 2004;273:199–200.
19. GTIN codes may be applied for at http://www.gs1uk.org/resources/help_support/Pages/ GS1numbersforbarcoding.aspx?gclid=CPT0_oiy9aMCFUg-4wodNG5X1w. Accessed January 2012.
20. Voss J. Launch of the X-factor for the visually impaired: the X-PIL. PIPA J. 2006;5:4–6.
21. Miller RA. Clinical decision support and electronic prescribing systems: a time for responsible thought and action. J Am Med Inform Assoc. 2005;12:403–9.
22. Goundrey-Smith S.J. For example, at Winchester & Eastleigh Hospitals Trust and Shrewsbury and Telford Hospitals Trust. Principles of Electronic Prescribing 1st Ed. Springer, London, p26, p29
23. Barker A, Kay J. Electronic prescribing improves patient safety – an audit. Hosp Pharm. 2007;14:225.
24. Gray S, Smith J. Practice report – electronic prescribing in Bristol. Healthc Pharm. 2004;(August):20–2.
25. Goddard J. Handheld computers in practice – clinical databases and intervention monitoring. In: Presented at the guild of Healthcare Pharmacists IT Interest Group seminar, Birmingham, 2003.
26. Barber N. Electronic prescribing – safer, faster, better? J Health Serv Res Policy. 2010;15 Suppl 1:64–7.
27. Lowery JC, Martin JB. Evaluation of healthcare software from a usability perspective. J Med Syst. 1990;14:17–29.

Chapter 2
Electronic Patient Records

Introduction

Healthcare professionals should maintain records of the patient care activities that they perform. While traditionally this has been a requirement from a medicolegal perspective, it is recognised that good record keeping supports evidence-based healthcare and facilitates audit and quality monitoring, which has become of increasing significance in many healthcare economies.

Over the last three decades, the use of patient medication record (PMR) systems by pharmacists in both hospitals and the community has become universal, and pharmacy professionals are familiar with the use of computerised records to support the dispensing process and provision of advice on medicines in their sphere of practice. However, in both primary care and secondary care, new pharmacy services and innovative ways of working are being developed, which require real-time access to electronic medical records for clinical decision making.

Quality of care and cost benefit monitoring is a pressing need in large economies, where there are considerable public health needs, and where the healthcare system is insurance-based, such as the United States. In recent years, with the increasing use of information technology to support patient records, there has been a focus on standard data recording as a means of facilitating consistency of care across a range of professional settings.

Furthermore, an increasingly multi-disciplinary approach to healthcare demands the use of patient records that are shared between different healthcare professionals. Electronic health record (EHR) systems enable this to happen.

However, electronic patient records contain sensitive, personal information about a patient's medical conditions and treatment, and this information is used to make important treatment decisions. In addition, electronic records have the capacity to be disseminated or accessed from different locations. For these reasons, the security and accessibility of the record are important issues in the development and use of electronic patient records, as is the question of who can or should contribute to the record and how they are identified.

S. Goundrey-Smith, *Information Technology in Pharmacy*,
DOI 10.1007/978-1-4471-2780-2_2, © Springer-Verlag London 2013

This chapter will explore the development of electronic health records (EHRs) in general, discuss the legal and design issues with EHRs, and describe how EHRs are used in pharmacy practice and how they can support other systems, and enable new initiatives in the profession. It will discuss issues such as access and sharing EHRs, subject (patient) access to records, specific record systems in the United States and United Kingdom, benefits of EHRs and how they might support pharmaceutical care.

Development of Electronic Patient Records

As discussed previously, the ability for healthcare professionals to store and retrieve electronic patient records has developed with the availability of solid state technology and computers that were small enough to be used in the office or clinical environment. Developments in communications and networking technology enabled electronic patient records to be shared within an enterprise – one particular hospital or healthcare provider – and this is commonplace today, in all major world economies. The use of enterprise-wide patient record systems enables a common subset of patient data to be used in all wards, clinics and departments of the provider organisation. However, the patient data available from the enterprise EHR or patient administration system (PAS) may be limited. It will only include patient demographic details (patient name, address, hospital/provider/insurance number etc) and no detailed information on clinical care. Consequently, it is common for enterprise EHR systems to be used as a feed of patient information for clinical or departmental systems which offer richer and more detailed functions – for example, e-prescribing, clinical decision support, clinical workflow and departmental management functions – but across a more limited domain. For example, in hospital pharmacies, many hospital pharmacy management systems have gained their feed of patient data from the enterprise PAS, and have used this to support specific pharmacy functionality such as labelling, decision support for drug interactions etc, pharmacy interventions, manufacturing worksheets etc.

In some situations, a rich medical record with details of diagnoses, medical history, clinical and treatment notes and care plan, will be available to health professionals in provider institutions across a geographical area, using a server and networked workstations. This is the case, for example, with US health maintenance organisation (HMO) records, such as Kaiser Permanente. Regional systems have been successfully developed in Sweden [1] and Italy [2], and the UK NHS IT initiatives have developed care records services in the UK. However, there are various political, professional and technical issues which can make the development of national centralised records services a slow process.

In addition to patient records on enterprise-based PAS and clinical systems, and national or regional centralised systems, there are also various private commercial providers of medical records software. The emphasis with these is that the individual, rather than the care provider or the state, takes ownership of, and responsibility for, the patient record, and this approach is being endorsed by some governments. Two such commercial EHR solutions are Google Health and MicroSoft Health Vault.

Legal and Professional Framework for EHRs

There are three important concepts in law (legal issues) concerning the generation and subsequent use of records of patient care and professional activity. They are:

* Confidentiality
* Consent
* Liability

These three concepts underpin the need to record medical observations and patient care interventions and are discussed here from the perspective of EHRs.

Confidentiality

The privacy of patient identifiable data (personal information) is governed in England by common law, by the Human Rights Act 1998 and the Data Protection Act 1998, and in the US by Federal law. Requirements for confidentiality in the UK NHS are described in the NHS Confidentiality Code of Practice [3]. Confidentiality is one of the key professional requirements for pharmacists and pharmacy technicians, as with other healthcare professions, and the principle of confidentiality is included in the standards issued by the General Pharmaceutical Council [4] in Great Britain and by other professional regulators.

Patients reasonably expect information collected in confidence in the context of a medical consultation to be stored securely, and treated in a confidential manner (not disclosed in an unauthorised manner). Health professionals, including pharmacists, therefore are said to have a duty of confidentiality, and are required to ensure that the confidentiality of patient information is safeguarded.

Where there is a need to transfer patient information from one care provider to another, professionals should ensure that the transfer of information takes place as securely as possible, in accordance with current information governance and security requirements. When deciding whether or not to share patient information, the pharmacy professional's duty of confidence should be weighed against the need for the continuity of effective care, and the consequences to the patient if the information is not shared, so that a decision is made that is in the patient's best interest.

There are some clearly defined circumstances where a pharmacy professional is required to share a patient information with a third party without the patient's consent [4], for example to assist the police with a criminal investigation.

Consent

In the UK, the Data Protection Act 1998 requires healthcare professionals to obtain a patient's consent to store information about them to support services provided, stating the purpose for which the information is being collected. The principle of consent is established in the General Pharmaceutical Council Professional Standards [5], and in those set by other professional regulators. Pharmacists should therefore seek explicit, informed consent from a patient to store and process information to support any pharmacy services, in situations where there is no other overriding legal requirement to keep records. In the UK, when a medicine is dispensed, pharmacy professionals are contractually obliged to make a record of the supply, and presentation of a prescription by a patient constitutes implied consent to this process. However, for any pharmacy service other than the dispensing of medicines, which requires an activity record containing patient identifiable information, patient consent must be sought to record and store their personal information.

Liability

As well as ensuring quality and continuity of care, records of patient care and treatment have traditionally played a major part in providing evidence of appropriate patient care in situations when allegations of negligence are made. This has not been a major issue for pharmacists in the past, but as pharmacists take on new roles, and provide clinically-focused professional services, they will need to make appropriate documentation of patient care interventions in order to account for their professional decision making.

Some pharmacists may be reluctant to document professional activity in case it is challenged by a patient or relative at a later time. However, pharmacists should bear in mind that there is an equal liability associated with not comprehensively recording details of care provided, and should ensure that information is recorded that will defend their professional decision-making.

The other major liability issue is concerning the use of information from standard records. If the information is available in a standard record, such as a centralized care record like the English summary care record (SCR), then it might be argued that the record must be accessed *every time* that a professional decision needs to be made, in order for the health professional to avoid liability. This a particular issue for pharmacists who are not working in clinic or office settings, and where records access is not easy, either for technical or feasibility reasons. For example, this issue has arisen in England with the proposed use of the NHS Summary Care Record by community pharmacists who would be working in busy dispensaries.

While specific services (for example, the English SCR) provide guidance for health professionals about liability associated with record use, the current consensus is that health professionals have a number of record sources available to them, and that they should use their professional judgment concerning the best record to access in each instance.

Information Governance and Data Sharing

In a healthcare environment where IT is increasingly used to produce a joined-up service across care settings, it is essential that community pharmacists, who may not be regarded as clinicians by the public, are seen to be handling patient information in a secure way when providing professional services.

This concern has been at the heart of the debate about community pharmacy access to the Summary Care Record, where some medical organisations and civil liberties campaigners have questioned the ability of pharmacists to handle sensitive patient information in what is seen as a "retail" environment. It is essential that community pharmacists fulfil their role as clinical professionals – but take on board the responsibilities that go with that role.

Information governance (IG) refers to the processes by which personal information is collected, managed, transmitted and used in a secure and confidential way in an organisation [6]. In the UK, the NHS Connecting for Health IG toolkit (www.igt. connectingforhealth.nhs.uk) for community pharmacy provides the pharmacy profession with guidance and a compliance framework to enable them to address these information management issues.

All patient information used by pharmacists, whether accessed from NHS services such as the Summary Care Record or stored in local or networked systems is subject to NHS information governance requirements in England. These requirements (currently 16 for community pharmacy in England) cover many aspects of good practice in information management and security and include, among others:

- Data transfer and sharing
- Risk assessment of data flows
- Staff Policies and Training
- Appointment of an IG lead
- Management of critical incidents
- Patient consent and awareness
- Use of mobile devices
- Physical security of hardware
- Use of mobile devices

Over the last few years, NHS Connecting for Health has rolled out IG requirements to various health professions in the UK – including GPs, pharmacists and dentists. Community pharmacies were required to undergo a baseline assessment by March 2010, and to have put into place a plan to achieve Level 2 IG toolkit compliance by March 2011.

Not only are the principles of IG essential for information security within individual organisations, they also have a key role in promoting intraoperability of systems, because it will assure the security of information transmitted between organisations in a standard format. It is clear from the UK government's recent Information Revolution consultation that IG requirements will support some of the UK Government's stated aims with healthcare IT, such as greater intraoperability and aggregation of outcomes data.

However, despite this clear requirement for IG compliance from an ethical and professional perspective, there are some pharmacists who regard IG requirements as another regulatory and bureaucratic burden that they have to work around. In the UK at present, the payor organisations, primary care trusts (PCTs), are responsible for implementing the IG agenda. Some PCTs have pushed for early pharmacy compliance with IG requirements – an approach that has not always been helpful. Some other PCTs have made little or no attempt to engage with the IG agenda, which has been equally unhelfpul.

IG provides a useful framework of information security for the professional duty of confidentiality in the electronic information age, and should be taken seriously by the pharmacy profession, in order to assure public trust and be in a good position to develop patient-centred services in a consistent way across different localities.

UK Health Records Standards Initiatives

In the UK, there have been a number of initiatives that have shaped the medical records and information management agenda. The Shared Record Professional Guidance (SRPG) project was commissioned by NHS Connecting for Health in England, and led by the Royal College of General Practitioners [7]. The aim of the project was to develop guidelines on the issues surrounding the use and governance of shared electronic patient record systems in primary care, and a range of professional bodies and stakeholder groups were engaged with this project. The project published a report which described includes 16 principles for record sharing in primary care. These were:

1. The success of shared records programmes should be measured alongside the operational characteristics of these programmes allowing evaluation of such systems in a wider context.
2. Joint guidance on record sharing should be produced and maintained collaboratively by professional regulatory bodies and representative organisations to ensure a multiprofessional approach to record quality, consistency and clarity
3. A community using a shared record system should establish clear governance rules and processes that ensure the clear allocation of responsibility and define the rules and mechanisms for its transfer.
4. Shared record systems should be designed to support the governance principles outlined in Principle 3.
5. Health professionals should have a shared responsibility for maintaining and assuring data quality in a shared record system.
6. The education and training of health professionals should enable them to meet their legal, ethical and professional responsibilities for using and managing shared record systems. This should form part of their ongoing professional development.
7. Semantic issues should be considered in the design and implementation of shared record systems so that meaning is preserved and must be sensitive to issues of language, interpretation and context.

8. Governance arrangements should be in place to deal with errors and differences of opinion in shared record systems.
9. Organisations should have the facility to update/correct erroneous information added to their records from other sources, (with the original information retained in the audit trail).
10. The content and provenance data should identify unambiguously the originator or editor of each entry in the shared record system.
11. Shared record systems should to be able to store and present information in styles that meet the particular user's needs.
12. Shared record systems should improve the quality and safety of care by facilitating communication and coordination between health professionals and informing best clinical practice.
13. Shared record systems should support structured communications between users.
14. Health organisations should be able to explain to patients who will have access to their shared record systems and must make information available to patients about such disclosures.
15. Health professionals should respect the wishes of those patients who object to particular information being shared with others providing care through a shared record system, except where disclosure is in the public interest or a legal requirement.
16. There should be an organisational guardian with clinical and information governance responsibilities for that organisation's shared record system in order to assure best practice is followed.

Another key issue with records standardization is that, in the past, records design has largely been the work of system suppliers, informatics specialists and some interested clinicians (largely doctors). However, for EHRs to be used universally in healthcare, there needs to be involvement of all healthcare professionals in record design, so that systems reflect the information needs and working processes of all healthcare professions.

In 2008, the UK NHS Connecting for Health (CfH) funded a project to broaden professional engagement in the development of clinical record standards, and to develop standards for the structure and content of health records. This project was led by the Royal College of Physicians (RCP), and engaged representatives from healthcare professional bodies, regulators, government agencies and other stakeholders. Following a national workshop and a consultation, the report "*Developing Standards for the Structure and Content of Health Records: Workshop Report*" was published in 2009 [8].

The report made the following recommendations:

- The rationale for professionally agreed record standards should be incorporated into pre- and post-registration educational curricula, and continuing professional development, as soon as possible.
- The standards agreed for the medical admission record, and handover and discharge communications, published by the RCP, should be disseminated widely and incorporated into the induction training of junior doctors as soon as possible.

- Healthcare professional bodies should work with stakeholders to take forward the development of standards for the structure and content of records appropriate to their own profession, specialty or discipline.
- This work should develop evidence and consensus based record standards for individual clinical specialties, care processes, and settings according to agreed priorities.

This initiative led not only to professional bodies taking steps towards formulating standards for record content which reflected their own disciplines, but also encouraged professional bodies to work together on record standards issues.

EHRs – Principles of Design and Use

What Is an EHR?

An electronic health record (EHR) may be defined as an information source in electronic form which contains identifiable information concerning a patient's medical care, and which is used to enable quality and continuity of care, and provide a record of care should subsequent queries arise.

The EHR may include, but is not restricted to:

- Diagnoses
- Medical History
- Allergies and ADRs
- Results of pathology and other tests
- Prescribing History

Systems Used for EPRs

A variety of electronic systems may be used to store EHRs. In pharmacy practice, these might include:

- Pharmacy systems or Patient Medication Record (PMR) systems for community pharmacy (see Chap. 6)
- GP systems and primary care medical record systems (see Chap. 5)
- National summary or emergency record services (e.g. the England Summary Care Record), which may be accessed via a pharmacy PMR system or by some other application.
- Other systems used by specific healthcare providers.

While this chapter will discuss the patient information within the systems, the detailed operation and workflow of pharmacy systems and GP systems will be considered in subsequent chapters. One or more of these systems may be available within a pharmacy or dispensary, depending on the type and affiliation of pharmacy (independent or multiple, separate organization or part of a medical practice).

Pharmacy professionals should exercise professional judgment concerning what information might be available from different systems, and should seek to make professional decisions with as much relevant information as is possible.

In multidisciplinary environments, the influence of pharmacy staff on the implementation and configuration of EHR systems may be limited. However, where possible, pharmacists should ensure that systems that they use comply with the principles of the UK NHS Care Record Guarantee [9] and other relevant information governance requirements, and industry standards. Pharmacy professionals also have a professional duty to ensure that EHR information is safeguarded from actions of non-pharmacist employers, which might compromise the integrity and confidentiality of the information.

EHR systems should provide appropriate access security, and should contain a comprehensive metadata set, including time and date stamps for each entry and an audit log of users making changes to records. The data fields on the EHR system should be adequate to provide the level of pharmaceutical care provided by the pharmacy.

Creation of EPRs

An EHR may be made available to pharmacists through a shared system such as a GP system, institutional medical record system or a national care record service, such as the English SCR. In this case, pharmacy professionals are not responsible for the creation of the record, although they are responsible for the safe access and appropriate use of the information in their sphere of practice.

However, pharmacy staff create a patient record de novo when patients seek a pharmacy service, and the pharmacy does not have access to a shared record.

When a patient brings a prescription or medicine order into a pharmacy to be dispensed, consent to the process of supply is implied and pharmacy contractual arrangements generally stipulate that a record of the supply must be kept on the PMR. Consent for the creation of a record relating to the supply of a medicine is therefore implied.

However, where a service is provided by the pharmacy which may or may not involve the supply of a medicine, then the patient must give informed consent to use of the service, which includes recording of patient information relating to the service on the EPR system. Therefore, if the patient presents for, or is recruited to, a pharmacy service in the community such as medicines review, management of long term conditions or smoking cessation, explicit consent must be given by the patient for their information to be recorded on the EPR system.

However, it is debatable how explicit, informed consent should be given to enable creation of an EHR. Health services, such as the UK NHS, have a legal duty to maintain adequate patient records, and patient records are routinely created by hospital staff according to the IG framework for the hospital or health trust, without the consent of the patient. Conversely, however, the provision of any pharmacy service in the community by a contractor body would require consent from the patient for creation of the record at the point where the service is provided.

In line with the Data Protection principles, pharmacy staff must ensure that patient information is relevant but not excessive. Where possible, to ensure completeness of the medication record, pharmacy staff should ensure that details of all medicines, including OTC and herbal medicines, are included in the EPR medication history.

Access to EHR Systems by Pharmacy Professionals

Pharmacy staff may access EHR systems for patient information in order to discharge their professional duties, in a way that is appropriate to their role and remit within the organisation.

There will be times when other pharmacy staff other than registered professionals will need to access the EHR system (for example technicians, assistants or counter staff), but they should do so under the supervision of a registered pharmacy professional.

Pharmacy staff must not access a patient record for any reason other than to enable provision of a pharmacy service. Use of the EHR for personal reasons would be unethical.

Where the EHR needs to be accessed for any other reason than the supply of a medicine – for example, to answer a patient query, or for an initial or follow up appointment for a pharmacy service – the patient's explicit consent must be obtained. This should be stated in any standard operating procedures (SOPs) for pharmacy services.

Consent for the use of the service and EHR should be sought in accordance with the appropriate legal requirements and professional standards for patient consent [5]. In England, an adult with the capacity to give consent or a child who understands the nature of the service (so-called Gillick competence) must give consent for use of the EHR. Consent for a young child should be given by a parent or guardian, and consent for an adult without capacity to give consent should be given by an appropriate person according to the Mental Capacity Act 2005.

Often, access to the record is requested by the representative of the patient, rather than the patient themselves. Pharmacy professionals should bear in mind that no-one can give consent on behalf of a competent adult and, depending on the circumstances, pharmacy professionals should consider whether it is necessary to speak to the patient directly. However, the pharmacy professional should act in the best interests of the patient in this situation, if it is not possible to speak to the patient directly.

Access to the patient's EHR by a health professional should be based on the professional's role, and whether they have a relationship with care with the patient. Thus, for a pharmacist to be able to access a patient's record, not only should the pharmacist be a registered pharmacist with an appropriate license to practice, they should also be the pharmacist who has been chosen or assigned to provide care to the patient concerned. These principles of role based access (RBAC) and legitimate relationship (LR) have been specifically developed in the English NHS care records service, and will be discussed in more detail later in this chapter.

There may be various access controls to systems holding EHRs within organisations. This may be a username and password system in many organizations, and these require a robust policy of routine password changes and timed log-outs to ensure that information is not viewed with someone else's log on ID. Biometric access (i.e. finger print or retinal scanning) is becoming more commonly used in many systems but is still too expensive to be scaleable in larger healthcare organizations. The UK national healthcare IT initiatives have a Smartcard and PIN system for gaining access to records services. The Smartcard and PIN, allows them access only to appropriate records, and to perform appropriate tasks in relation to those records. The process for obtaining a Smartcard involves the healthcare professional proving identity beyond reasonable doubt, and then they are given appropriate access privileges based on their NHS role. The NHS has had to ensure that there are appropriate procedures for Smartcard issue and maintenance, both for healthcare practitioners and students/trainees. This must be based on verification of identity, just as for other NHS staff and contractors.

The issue and maintenance of Smartcards for healthcare professionals is controlled by a Registration Authority (RA) in each area. The RA is an NHS body, usually the PCT (payor) organization. At present only NHS organisations can set up a Registration Authority and this has two implications:

- RAs need to work jointly with educational establishments to manage the process of identity checking and issuing of Smartcards to students and placement trainees.
- Non-NHS bodies may not act as a RA, even if they have the resources and the governance framework to do so. This is of particular importance to pharmacy; for some time, large pharmacy multiples have wanted to set themselves up as RAs, in order to better manage the issuing and use of Smartcards held by employee pharmacists, wherever they are based. There is a sound operational argument for pharmacy multiples to be designated RAs.

Liability for Record Use

Pharmacy professionals are responsible for the completeness, accuracy and timeliness of information on EHR systems used in the pharmacy setting, if they are able to make entries to the record.

If a pharmacy professional makes a professional decision in good faith based on information in the EPR that is subsequently found to be inaccurate, they should not be liable for any unintended clinical consequence. However, pharmacy professionals would be expected to be alert to any obvious errors or discrepancies in the record, according to their qualifications and experience.

If a pharmacy professional identifies an error in an existing EHR, and they have write access to the record, they should correct the error and amend the record appropriately, if they have the correct information to do so. If the pharmacy professional does not have write access to the record, they should inform the record's originator.

As mentioned, a pharmacy may have one or more EHR systems available. Pharmacy professionals should use the most appropriate information sources to support their professional decision making. Pharmacy staff should review any information that may be feasibly accessed in order to reach a professional decision, according to their professional judgment.

However, pharmacists should bear in mind that if they chose not to view a patient's records stored on the PMR or not to contact a doctor to ask for the medical records to be checked then, were the patient then to come to harm or subsequently complain because of an issue that arose as a result, it might be difficult to defend the case.

Subject Access to EHRs

Under the UK Data Protection legislation, the subject of any personal information has a right of access to that information. In the UK, the patient's right of access to their medical records is established in the NHS Constitution [10] and the Information Commissioner's Office provides guidance about subject access to patient records [11]. In addition, the Royal College of General Practitioners has issued guidance on providing patients with access to their medical records, which covers legal and ethical background; security, registration and authentication; guidance for health professionals writing records that can be shared with the patient; self management and shared decision making; test results; the patient sharing the record with someone else; third party data; psychiatric and mental health data; children; and responding to issues of accuracy and interpretation identified by the patient.

Evidence from the medical profession suggests that access to EHRs by patients has benefits in patient care, and does not lead to increased litigation [12]. So-called triadic consulting where both the clinician and the patient view the EHR on the computer screen during the course of the consultation is common in many areas of medicine [13].

The presence of a consulting room/area in pharmacies for the conduct of medicine reviews (medicines use reviews (MURs)) and other pharmacy services, with a workstation in the consulting room enables pharmacists to discuss medicines with a patient, with the EHR available to view for both parties. However, it should be remembered that there may be occasions where the pharmacist will need to view the patient's record prior to a consultation, without the patient being present.

If the patient identifies an error in their record when viewing the EHR, then the pharmacy professional should use their professional judgment to take appropriate steps to correct the record, validating any new information from the patient, and liaising with the patient's GP as necessary.

Viewing the EHR

The availability of the EHR on a workstation in the <u>consulting room</u> has made it easy for the health professional and the patient to view a patient's record during the course of the consultation, although healthcare professionals may need to develop consultations skills that enable them to use an EHR as part of the consultation in an appropriate way.

Pharmacists are increasingly providing a wider range of healthcare services to patients, and many community pharmacies have consultation areas on their premises. However, while some of these consulting areas may be specific, separate rooms for the purposes of patient consultation, others may be no more than booths or kiosks offering little privacy away from the dispensary or retail space.

While is to be hoped that all community pharmacies invest in adequate consultation rooms, there may be circumstances where space and resources limit the facilities that can be made available. Nevertheless, pharmacists will need to consider how an EHR workstation may be appropriately used in the consulting room, and how the security of the information available on the workstation can be maintained.

Pharmacy managers should take steps to ensure that a patient's record is only on screen for the duration of the consultation and that systems are in place to ensure that the workstation cannot be accessed in an unauthorised manner when the consultation room is not in use.

Sharing of Data

There may be occasions when data on a patient from an EHR system used by pharmacists may need to be shared with another healthcare professional or provider to provide the most appropriate care for the patients. Where a shared record system is established, and the other healthcare professional is a system user, this issue presents no specific difficulties. However, if the patient's information is to be shared with healthcare professionals and providers from external organizations, pharmacists would need to consider how patients are advised of the need to share data with third parties.

When <u>sharing patient data</u> with other health professionals, pharmacy professionals should ensure that appropriate <u>confidentiality</u> and data security measures are in place, in accordance with <u>information governance</u> requirements (for example when sending faxes). While pharmacists have a duty of confidentiality, the need for absolute patient confidentiality should be balanced with the need for the continuity of effective care, and the consequences to the patient if the information is not shared because the patient's consent could not be obtained.

Under the UK NHS CfH Information Governance requirements for pharmacy, pharmacy organisations should make patients aware of what data are collected and stored about them at the pharmacy (or available to the pharmacy), and with whom this data might be shared. This process would be via an information sheet that is available at the pharmacy, and given to new patients coming to the pharmacy.

If a patient's information needs to be shared with a health professional or provider not mentioned in the patient awareness leaflet, the patient's explicit consent should be sought to share the data.

Pharmacy staff should be aware that there are some statutory situations where a patient's data may be disclosed to a third party without the patient's consent, for example, cooperation with the police in a criminal investigation.

Use of Data for Purposes Other Than That for Which It Was Collected

Patient data on EHR systems should be used only for the provision of pharmacy services and for identification of individuals eligible for pharmacy services under the supervision of a pharmacist. Patient data on EHR systems must not be used inappropriately or in an unprofessional manner.

The use of EHRs in the pharmacy must be in line with appropriate legal requirements, information governance arrangements and professional standards. Data from EHRs must not be used for commercial purposes, other than the provision of pharmacy services. Furthermore, EHR data should not be used for research purposes without the appropriate patient consent and ethics approvals being secured from the appropriate authority.

Business Continuity

Pharmacy organisations using EHRs routinely for patient care should satisfy themselves that system suppliers and other IT support services have appropriate business continuity arrangements in place to ensure that, if systems fail, there is an appropriate level of EPR access to ensure the safety and quality of patient care.

There is a requirement for business continuity in the England Information Governance requirements for pharmacy, for which more detailed guidance is currently being prepared.

Archiving and Destruction of Records

EPRs must be retained by organisations in accordance with legal requirements for records retention, and local records management policies. The usual UK legal requirement is that personal health records should be retained for 8 years after the date of last treatment/record access.

Electronic Health Record Initiatives

Large, integrated health record systems have been installed by healthcare maintenance organisations (HMOs) in the United States, such as the Veterans' Administration (VA) and Kaiser Permanente (KP). These systems provide a medical record, with supporting functions, to support medical centres across large regions. These systems will store patient data and also support medication records, clinical decision support, test results and electronic billing and claims. With a common technical infrastructure and within a single HMO, the use of these systems may be critical for ensuring the quality of care and appropriate resource management in patients with long term conditions [14]. However, to date, there has been little research to quantify the benefits of EHRs to support integrated healthcare delivery by US HMOs.

Graez et al. [15] studied the effect of EHRs on the coordination of healthcare in the KP north California scheme, and found that clinicians with 6 months or more experience of using EHRs were more likely to report timely access to complete medical information, and a broader consensus on treatment goals among clinicians involved in a patient's case. These findings are likely to lead to a reduction in the number of medication related errors in this environment.

In a study of the KP Ohio scheme, Khoury [16] indicated that the system improved compliance with clinical guidelines, improved classification of asthma patients, provided streamlined electronic billing and reduced operating costs for the organisation.

A study of clinician attitudes to the North-western KP programme, based at Portland, Oregon (Marshall and Chin [17]) showed that clinicians perceived an improvement in the quality of patient care with the use of the EHR with increased ability to coordinate care with different departments and to detect medication errors, and improved timeliness of referrals and test results reporting.

Nevertheless, not all experiences of EHRs for integrated care in HMOs have been positive. In a study of the KP Hawaii scheme, Scott et al. [18] found that the process of EHR implementation was not straightforward. They found that:

- There were software design issues that increased resistance to the adoption of the system.
- The system reduced clinicians' productivity, especially in the early stages of system implementation, an observation that has been made with some electronic prescribing systems.

- The system required clarification of clinical roles and responsibilities, which caused some concerns for clinicians and other staff.

It is possible that some of these implementation issues could be surmounted with an appropriate change management process.

Also in the US, systems have been developed which provide a centralised, aggregated record of medicines information relating to both prescribing and pharmacy activity. The Regenstrief medication hub [19] has been developed in the US to combine patient prescribing records with pharmacy claims data, to produce a complete and integrated medication record, which can then be used to support electronic prescribing. This system also provides benefit eligibility data on treatments and can therefore be used to provide formulary control. The need for an integrated medicines record is discussed in greater depth in Chap. 6.

The English Summary Care Record (SCR) has been developed for use in unscheduled care settings (for example, A&E or out of hours medical care) when the detailed electronic care record is unavailable. The SCR content has been uploaded from GP summary information. The SCR provides four key elements of information – diagnosis, current medications, allergies, and adverse reactions and, in some areas, other aspects of the GP record. The Summary Care Record has been piloted extensively in order to test both the clinical utility of the information displayed and also the procedure for discussing and recording the patient's permission to view SCR data.

The Summary Care Record contains the following information:

1. Allergies.
2. Adverse reactions.
3. Acute prescriptions in last 6 months.
4. Current repeat prescriptions.
5. Discontinued repeat prescriptions in last 6 months.
6. *May* also contain additional information such as diagnoses or patient preferences.

The SCR may also contain additional information such as significant medical history. The SCR offers particular benefits for unscheduled care – for example A&E departments will be able to view a patient's record to assist with the emergency treatment of that patient, for whom they may have no information. The SCR has been shown to be of considerable value for medicines reconciliation by pharmacy staff when patients are admitted to hospital, and has been used for this at the Bolton Hospitals [20]. It is now being piloted to assess its benefits in community pharmacy.

The SCR is a form of EHR and the general principles described above apply to its use in a pharmacy setting. However, the SCR has specific rules and concepts, which will be briefly discussed here. The use of the SCR in pharmacy settings is in its infancy in England and, while a number of localities have used the SCR, official pilot studies will be required to fully understand the practical use of the SCR and any procedural issues associated with it in a pharmacy context. The SCR is one of several possible sources of medicines information available to the pharmacist, and its use should be considered in the context of the other sources of information available to a patient.

For further information please see:

http://www.connectingforhealth.nhs.uk/systemsandservices/scr

Access to a patient's Summary Care Record is governed by the permission to view model developed by NHS Connecting for Health. The patient's permission must be sought to view that patient's Summary Care Record and this process is based on six principles:

1. The explanation to a patient, as part of seeking permission to view, should be simple, straightforward, honest and appropriately communicated.
2. A patient's permission should be sought by the care setting wishing to view their Summary Care Record.
3. Care settings should be explicit about the scope of permission being sought i.e. who is being given permission, for how long and in what context.
4. The scope of permission obtained must be recorded.
5. Before setting the "not to be asked in future" consent status for a patient, the user must be sure of the patient's wishes in terms of scope of this permission.
6. Permission to view does not apply where the patient is unable to give permission to view, and the clinician acts in the patient's best interests.

Pharmacists must therefore seek permission to view from the patient for each episode of care for they wish to access the patient's SCR. However, there are a number of issues that affect pharmacies concerning permission to view. An "episode of care" may be activity-based, for example, the dispensing of one prescription or the installments of a repeat prescription. Alternatively, the episode of care may be time-based – for example, permission to view for all pharmacy activities for that patient in a 6 month period. The activity-based approach is problematic as pharmacy staff would need to ask patients repeatedly for permission to view for different activities taking place concurrently, and would be required to not use information that they already knew from the SCR for a second activity, if that permission were not given.

A time-based approach to episodes of care is therefore more practical, although pharmacists would need to identify suitable means for recording permission and put in place a system to allow for updating of permission to view when the period ends, if a designated time period is agreed.

The other issue for pharmacies is how permission to view would work if a patient received services from a pharmacy multiple, and could present at two or more of its local branches. Permission may apply to more than one branch, but the pharmacist requesting the permission to view would need to explicitly request this, and the patient would need to fully understand the scope of the permission to view that they have granted.

As already mentioned, a clinician needs to have a legitimate relationship with a patient in order to view a patient's clinical information. That is to say that only healthcare staff actually involved in the patient's care can view their clinical information.

The SCR conventions define several types of LR, but only two LR types are relevant to the use of the SCR in community pharmacy. They are:

- Patient Self Referral LR – created when a patient presents themselves for treatment to an individual or a workgroup (a team, or set of teams, that work together to provide a service to patients) and which has role separation and lasts for 26 weeks. Role separation means that one person sets up the LR and another accesses the clinical information e.g. call handler and clinician or pharmacy worker and pharmacist.
- Clinician Self Claimed LR – created for a single user accessing the SCR without a workgroup or role separation and therefore without validation from a second party, which lasts 5 days.

A concern that many English pharmacists have is how the information provided on the SCR relates to that which they will have available on their pharmacy system. Pharmacists will be confident with the patient medication record information on the pharmacy system/PMR, but there will be times when the use of a national service such as the SCR will supplement the local information available on the pharmacy system. For example, using the SCR may help to resolve a discrepancy between the pharmacy system and the prescription, or between the pharmacy system and the patient's recollection.

Pharmacists have also raised the issue of transfer of information from the SCR into local IT systems. Transfer of information into local systems by cutting and pasting may be beneficial to patients. However, if information from the SCR is placed into a local system, there is no mechanism to ensure that the information is updated. Furthermore, the owners of the local system are then required to maintain the security of their local system in a manner comparable to the national system.

In Wales, the Individual Health Record will be created from the GP summary, and is available to doctors and nurses routinely in out of hours services, and is being used by pharmacists at the Medical Admissions Unit at the Royal Gwent Hospital.

The Individual Health Record contains the following details:

- Name, address and contact details
- Details of current GP practice
- Record of current and recent medication
- Medical problems from GP consultations
- Recorded allergies
- Results of any recent tests – for example, blood tests and x-rays

Only the last 2 years of medication history and 1 year of test results will be shown.

As with the English Summary Care Record, patients need to give consent to allow a health professional to access their record, and there is an opt-out system for patients who do not want to have an Individual Health Record.

The Scotland Emergency Care Summary (ECS) contains the following information:

• Name
• Date of Birth
• CHI Number (NHS Scotland identifier)
• GP Surgery details
• Allergies and ADRs
• Prescribing History

The ECS is viewable by doctors and nurses at out of hours centres, A&E departments and also by NHS 24 staff. Pharmacists have been able to gain access to ECS information through patient contact with NHS 24. In the near future, the ECS will be tested for medicines reconciliation by hospital pharmacists.

The ECS is extracted from the GP record and, as with other national health records in Great Britain, patient consent is required every time the record is accessed. Patients may opt out of the scheme by contacting their GP surgery.

Benefits of EHRs

EHRs provide a number of benefits (benefits of EHRs) to healthcare professionals in their professional practice and in delivery of healthcare services. These include:

• Enabling record security – depending on the design of the system, EHRs are likely to be more secure that paper records.
• Structured content of the record – the record may be structured in such a way as to support each professional activity in the healthcare workflow. Thus, in a GP system, the record content can be displayed in a structured screen to aid the GP consultation process.
• Provision of decision support tools – the availability of the patient record in an electronic format means that electronic decision support tools can be made available in an interruptive or non-interruptive manner at the point where information is entered onto the record.
• Patient record information is legible and may be used to support other IT applications.
• Improved access to patient information for healthcare professionals authorized to view a patient record.

Because of these features, EHRs have the potential to reduce adverse drug events and improve patient outcomes by their effects on the quality of care. However, the results of studies on the clinical benefits of EHRs are mixed. In a transfer of care study, Boockvar et al. [21] concluded that there was no difference between patients with an EHR and non-EHR patients, in terms of the number of medication-related discrepancies in the records, and that specialist tools would be required as part of the record system to facilitate medicines review. Indeed, Hurdle et al. [22] noted how a large number of adverse events relating to medication remained undetected within a Veterans' Administration (VA) EHR system in the US, despite a prospective chart review study. In any case, even if decision support tools within an EHR are effective, there may not be an obvious link between appropriate decision support alerts and positive patient outcomes. This was observed by Smith et al. [23], in a study on the Kaiser Permanente, North-Western system, where alerts were found to reduce the prescribing of potentially contraindicated agents (e.g. tricyclic antidepressants) in the elderly, but the effect of the alerts on patient outcomes and morbidity was not clear. In a US study, Orrico [24] noted discrepancies between the EHR system record and actual medicine use. It was common for medicines to be recorded on the EHR, but no longer taken by the patient. They indicated that medicine stop/review dates would be helpful to prevent this situation, and that a system of medicines reconciliation and review would be beneficial.

However, the use of structured data within an EHR system has the potential to identify cohorts of patients systematically where intervention may have positive health benefits. In a study looking at the identification of adverse events relating to amlodipine in UK general practice, Mohamed et al. [25] concluded that primary care prescribing databases could easily be used to identify ADRs by looking at cohorts of patients where a medicine has been discontinued. In a data study of 61,251 patients in two US outpatient settings, Buck et al. [26] demonstrated that EHRs could be used to identify potentially inappropriate medication (PIM); they found that female sex, polypharmacy (≥6 medicines) and multiple clinic visits were key determinants in identifying patients with PIM. While these factors themselves are well recognised in the literature as pointers to poor prescribing, the EHR system automates the search process by which patients can be identified. The use of EHRs for screening patients for medication related problems was also demonstrated by Roten et al. [27] in a Swiss clinical pharmacy study with 501 patients. They found that the EHR efficiently identified drug related problems in 64.7 % of the 501 patients.

In an Australian study, Berbatis and Sunderland [28] looked at the impact of linked EHRs for the prevention of diversion of pseudoephedrine for abuse purposes. They found that the use of EHRs to monitor supplies of drugs from a number of sources was an effective way of dealing with the pseudoephedrine problem and could be used for other drugs of abuse too.

Frenzel [29] has further conjectured that EHRs could be structured with disease management in mind, and could be used to teach pharmacy students disease management activities, and help them to develop patient care skills.

A benefit of a patient's EHR being available in a controlled electronic format is the potential for direct patient access to the record via a web portal. In the UK and other countries, more patients want to be able to view their medical records and the UK Royal College of General Practitioners has produced guidance to help doctors deal with patient requests for access [12]. However, there is little documented experience of remote patient access to EHRs to date. In a telephone survey of citizens of seven European countries, Santana et al. [30] found that the use of the internet for communications between patients and healthcare professionals was still rare. A Swedish study of a web portal to make medication record information available to patients [31] found that users of the service appreciated having their medication information available to them on the web, and the authors recognized that there was a need to make more patients aware of the service. However, there may be social and cultural factors affecting the uptake of online access to medical records. Roblin et al. [32] compared use of the KP Georgia scheme personal health record (web access to health records) in white and African Americans, and found that fewer African Americans than white Americans used the internet access scheme, and that differences in education, income and internet access did not account for this difference.

A Nuffield expert report on EHR use [33] indicated that EHRs had the potential to be transformative technology, which could provide end-to-end healthcare and change ways of working. However, the importance of EHRs was about providing clinical benefits, not just managing patient information. The authors highlighted that, while institutional systems in the US, such as VA and KP had the potential to deliver clinical and organisational benefits, there was a lack of evidence on the economic benefits of these systems. The potential benefits of EHR systems for the management of long term conditions are well recognized by governments and policy-makers. Barrett and Jennings [34] reported that the goal of the Canadian Health Infoway programme was to ensure that 50 % of Canadians had a electronic health record by 2010, including a prescribing history, allergy alerts and drug interactions, but this has not been fully achieved. Likewise, the purpose of the meaningful use initiative in the United States was to encourage more widespread use of EHRs by HMOs and providers, to harness patient safety and quality of care benefits. However, a study by Linder et al. [35], looking at the prescribing of antibiotics in response to a EHR respiratory infection dashboard, indicated that the meaningful use initiative in itself was not sufficient to improve care quality, and that improvements in clinical practice were required.

A 2009 report on the impact of EHRs [36] looked at a number of European systems and concluded that, with EHRs, the socioeconomic gain usually outweighed the costs eventually, but that the benefits realization phase was often quite long, in the order of 4–11 years following system implementation.

Clinical Pathways and Content

As well as explicit workflow decision support tools, EHR systems may be used to provide electronic care pathways, where the user is directed along a particular care pathway for a patient, based on the workflow of the system. The NHS in England has been developing care pathways since the1990s, but progress with the development of electronic care pathways has been slow. A good approach would be the prioritization of electronic care pathways for those areas where there is a substantial national consensus on paper-based care pathways, e.g. stroke, diabetes and falls. A useful UK initiative is the Map of Medicine, which provides evidence-based treatment pathways for a range of disease areas [37].

Related to the development of electronic care pathways is the development of electronic templates for clinical assessment tools for use by healthcare professionals in provider organisations. The templates will enable staff to directly record assessment data into the patient's EHR. Once recorded electronically, the assessment data can be used by all healthcare staff involved in that service user's direct care, and for secondary purposes, e.g. clinical research, audit, performance management and commissioning. In the UK, these tools have been developed by various healthcare professions, most notably occupational therapists, but the use of these in pharmacy practice is still in its infancy because pharmacists have traditionally not conducted their consultations in an office environment with a workstation at the point of consultation.

While various software tools have been developed to support pharmacist consultations (within and beyond pharmacy management systems) for new pharmacy services, it is to be hoped that there would be more standardization of clinical assessment tools and content to support pharmacist activity in future. This may involve the adoption of clinical content or workflows developed in a multidisciplinary way, but there will be a need to develop material specifically to support pharmacist working processes.

The following elements are needed to develop authoritative and useful clinical content:

- An appropriate sponsor, e.g. healthcare professional body
- Widespread use and best practice recommendation for a specific assessment purpose
- No copyright or licensing issue for use in relevant health provider organizations.

Once clinical content has been developed and endorsed by professional bodies, it can then be adopted by suppliers of EHR and other systems.

Optimisation of EHRs for Pharmaceutical Care

Hospital pharmacists in the UK have undertaken some important pioneering work in creating pharmaceutical care record templates and recording systems to support their field of practice [38, 39]. However, while a number of centres around the UK have developed record templates, this work has not been undertaken consistently around the country and a national standard for pharmaceutical care has long been sought by clinical pharmacists.

The development of a pharmaceutical care record standard has the potential to provide the following benefits:

- Providing an agreed standard for format and content of pharmaceutical care records, which is patient-centred and therefore independent of care setting and area of pharmacy practice. This may be used as a foundation for the development of innovative services.

- Promoting a unified approach to pharmaceutical care and intervention recording across the pharmacy profession, and therefore improve communications across the profession.
- Provision of a standard to support professional teaching and development.
- Increasing awareness outside the profession of the contribution that pharmacists make to patient care.
- Improving communications between pharmacists, other healthcare professionals and patients.
- Providing a standard for future development of IT systems in medicines management.
- Providing a foundation against which key outcome measures may be determined.

However, the development and adoption of an agreed standard for data content and format in recording pharmaceutical care and pharmacy interventions highlights a number of important issues that would need to be acknowledged or addressed in the development of any record standard.

Firstly, any standard produced for pharmaceutical care would need to support aspects of care of particular importance to pharmacy (e.g. formulation types, compliance and use of compliance aids), but would need to be consistent with the work of other healthcare professions in this field. In the UK, the most prominent standard for record keeping on medicines is Royal College of Physicians medical records standards for admission and discharge.

Secondly, a standard for record keeping will highlight pharmacy practice more which could then be open to scrutiny. While a culture of record keeping and recording details of care provided has been in place in the medical profession for many years, this is a new concept for many pharmacists. A standard care record for pharmacy practice may therefore be perceived as a threat by some pharmacists, and they may need training in note-taking and maintaining records of interventions. Work in other professions has shown that failure to make records can be detrimental to patient care and professional accountability.

Thirdly, some pharmacists have been routinely maintaining records of interventions made and care provided in their specialist areas of practice for some years now. The adoption of a standard pharmaceutical care record will need to take into account and affirm the good work that these pharmacists are already doing.

Applications of EHRs for Pharmacists

EHRs of different forms may have a number of applications for pharmacists in their professional practice. These include:

- When dispensing prescriptions to check for interactions, contraindications and allergy status. It is recognised that PMR systems already provide functions to check allergy status and interactions.

- Supporting self care and promoting healthy lifestyles – knowing what (other) medication a patient is taking.
- For conducting medicines reviews.
- For conducting medicines reconciliation at the point of hospital admission.
- During a medicines use review (MUR) to verify and compare medications currently being prescribed for the patient and their allergy status.
- When supplying over the counter (OTC) medication from the pharmacy.
- When dispensing private prescriptions.
- When dispensing an emergency supply (at the request of the patient) to allow the pharmacy professional to verify the name, form, strength and dose of medication previously had by the patient.
- When recording details of interventions made by the pharmacist concerning a prescription or over the counter medicine sale. The Royal Pharmaceutical Society of Great Britain has previously issued guidance on the recording of interventions [40] giving advice on when to record interventions, where to record interventions and how long to retain intervention records for. However, while the guidance gives outline advice on what information to record, this is not covered in detail.

The Content of a Pharmaceutical Care Record

The best approach to developing the requirements for a standard EHR designed for use for a particular healthcare professional practice is to consider the scenarios that the healthcare professional faces in their professional practice. This will enable the development of a use case for each scenario, and for the specific information requirements around the scenario or activity to be understood. These scenarios should describe the care activities for the patient – so, from a pharmacy perspective, the process planning to design the EHR should be focussed on the care of the patient, rather than the supply of the product.

This would mean that:

- An outline as to the type of processes and formatting required could be identified.
- The required data items would be clearly identifiable from the scenarios described.
- The correct set of patient information would follow the patient from one care setting or scenario to another.

Each pharmacy practice scenario described should be analysed by asking the questions:

- Who?
- Where?
- When?
- What?

This approach would ensure that the pharmaceutical care processes are fully understood. Subsequent implementation of a well-designed pharmaceutical care record would ensure that the pharmacy team providing care is able to identify and meet the pharmaceutical needs of a patient and take responsibility for delivering the appropriate care.

A pharmaceutical care record should take into account the interdisciplinary care of the patient. The pharmacist may therefore also want to know and record:

- What other HCP are involved in their care (are any professionals not involved who should be?)
- Recommendations made by other healthcare team members
- Referrals made to other healthcare team members arising from disease monitoring
- Any professional concerns that have been recorded – whether they have been followed up or alerted to other professionals (e.g. social care)?

The boundaries between healthcare and social care may not be clearly delineated within a healthcare economy, and professional bodies and policy makers may need to make scope decisions concerning the adoption and use of record systems.

Appendix B gives a suggested domain map for a standard pharmaceutical care record. A pharmaceutical care record would therefore need to have the following basic elements:

1. Patient Demographics – sufficient to identify the correct patient beyond reasonable doubt.
2. Patient Details – age, weight
3. GP Details
4. Social Information
5. Previous Medical History
6. ADRs/Allergies
7. Current/Recent Medication
8. Tests & Investigations
9. Pharmacist Recommendation – medicine and counselling
10. Referral Information
11. Recent referrals, new referral

A key assumption of the process is that all information recorded is date, time and user stamped, in order that an audit trail of care could be established.

Pharmaceutical care records should support the following situations.

Medicines Reviews

Pharmaceutical care records should support the process of medicine review in an iterative manner. There are two distinct types of review scenario:

(a) Medicines Use Review (MUR) (primary care based review and probably a sub-set of a clinical review) (a specific remunerated service in the English pharmacy content)
(b) Clinical review (broader more in-depth review).

MURs can happen without an appointment, and therefore can be opportunistic. An MUR can be conducted in response to an intervention, or to determine if a full clinical review is warranted. With an MUR, information on medication use is obtained from the patient, to initiate a two way dialogue concerning concordance, to determine the patient's views and beliefs about their medicines. MURs are practically and socially based. Patients need to consent for an MUR to be conducted and communication to GPs or onwards as necessary. For medicines reviews, a pharmaceutical care record should be able to record reason for the review, consent to the review, comments concerning specific medicines, and provide decision support for specific medicines.

Medicines Reconciliation

The process of medicines reconciliation is where a pharmacist or pharmacy technician reviews a patient's medication when the patient is admitted to hospital or other healthcare institution, by taking a full medication history from the patient. The medication history taken from the patient is then compared with the actual medicines brought in by the patient, and available medication records, in order to ascertain exactly what medicines a patient has been prescribed and what medicines they are actually taking. The availability of a centralised medication record from the patient's usual physician is an important part of establishing an exact medical history and therefore ensuring that (a) important medicines that the patient has been taking are not inadvertently omitted, or (b) that the patient does not suffer adverse effects from being given a medicine in hospital that was prescribed but was not actually taken prior to admission. Consequently, centralised systems such as HMO systems in the US and summary records such as the SCR, ECS and IHR in the UK have an important role to play to enable medicines reconciliation in hospitals. Smith [20] has reported the use of the SCR for medicines reconciliation at Bolton Hospital, UK. The use of the SCR for medicines reconciliation provided the following benefits:

• The system provided an accurate source of up to date information.
• The system was accessible outside the opening hours of doctor's surgeries/offices, and meant that doctors did not have to spend time responding to routine medication enquiries.
• There was an improvement in patient safety and quality of care.
• The system provided an auditable record of access to patient data.

Similar benefits have been reported by users of the Scottish ECS and the Welsh IHR. In addition, specialist software has been developed to enable local medicines

Fig. 2.1 Care process for
treatment of long-term
conditions

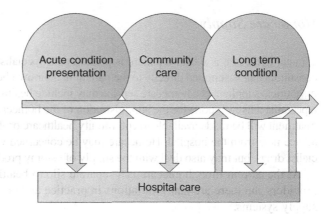

reconciliation. Schnipper et al. [41] conducted a quantitative study on an electronic
medicines reconciliation system, and found that its use led to a small decrease in
medicines discrepancies, from 1.44 per patient, to 1.05 per patient.

Shared Care

This encompasses medicines that are managed jointly between different elements of
the NHS. It thus covers medicines that are wholly secondary care managed as well
as those that are managed jointly, and may also include community-based services
(e.g. family planning etc). These are medicines for which an incorrect assumption
that the hospital is managing the monitoring, prescribing etc is made when this may
or may not be the case.

The pharmaceutical care record requirements for this situation should therefore facilitate the sharing of information about care in another setting (formal and informal), and
identify specific responsibilities for care, as well as manage the transfer of care process.

Care across interfaces can cover the following clinical situations – chemotherapy,
epoeitin, renal dialysis, anti TNF agents, pharmacist clinics, 'red' drugs – hospital
only, pumps, implants, specialist imports, CIVAS items and various others.

Long Term Condition Management

The pharmaceutical care record should facilitate exchange of information and continuity of care between acute treatment settings and chronic care of long term conditions. It
should be able to provide support to the pharmacist who takes on responsibility for
monitoring and support of, and supplementary prescribing for, patients with long-term
conditions in the community. Figure 2.1 summarises the possible relationship between
acute condition, community care and long term condition management in primary care.
Pharmaceutical care records should be designed with this or a similar process in mind.

Homecare Supply

Clinical homecare is where a patient is prescribed a specialist treatment by a hospital consultant that is supplied directly to the patient in their own home by a homecare pharmaceutical supplier. The homecare service may include healthcare professional support (specialist nurse support) for the administration of the homecare product. Details of the treatment will be made available to community healthcare professionals via a discharge advice note from the hospital. Homecare may be concerned with the provision of specialist drugs, but may also deal with the supply of ostomy products or enteral feeds.

At the current time, homecare is a separate silo to healthcare provided by other providers and there are many variations in practice and governance with homecare supply systems.

There are a number of successful outcome criteria for a homecare service:

• Provision of a safe, effective homecare treatment service
• There are good communications and all healthcare professionals involved in patient care know what has been supplied within homecare arrangements.
• Continuity of cover of homecare supplies
• Systems in place for updating homecare records in a timely and accurate way

Appliances

Medical devices and appliances may be supplied by pharmacists but also by other suppliers and delivery services (e.g. appliance contractors). A wide variety of people, other than the patient and the lead healthcare professional, may be involved with the use of a device, or need to know about a device. These might include: practice nurses, specialist nurses, carers and relatives, nutritionists and dieticians (stoma etc), physiotherapists, occupational therapists, other AHP, teaching staff (with children and young people) and various others.

Devices might include:

• Ostomy bags and consumables
• Catheters
• Dressings
• Nebulisers

The usual pattern is that diagnosis, surgery or acute treatment occurs in hospital and first fitting or use of the device takes place in hospital (either before discharge or at a subsequent outpatient appointment, if the device/appliance needs to be ordered).

Once the patient is discharged, the appliance or device may be used in any community setting. Routine assessments and supplies of devices will take place during working hours, but there may be out-of-hours queries (patient use queries, emergency cases or complications). Specialist suppliers may take over patient supplies on a longer term basis, and the danger is that the patient's progress is not then reviewed by the pharmacist or other healthcare professional.

The success criteria for the supply and use of devices and appliances are:

• Seamless provision of the correct device and ancillary equipment
• Minimum waste
• Single point of contact for the patient
• Underlying condition is controlled with minimum complications
• Emergencies/unexpected situations can be dealt with easily

Patient Group Direction (PGD) Supply

The Patient Group Direction (PGD) is a means of supplying or administering a prescription only medicine without an individual prescription. While a record of supply should be made, the PGD supply can take place on a confidential basis (e.g. with Emergency Hormonal Contraception). The purpose of PGDs is to widen patient access to treatment in areas where there are specific public health needs.

PGD supply may take place in a number of settings, for example, the patient's home, a walk in clinic or a residential home, not just in the pharmacy.

Public Health and Screening

Pharmacists may be involved in local public health or disease screening initiatives. These initiatives are designed to improve health and screen for disease in hard-to-reach groups of the population or people who do not go to see their GP.

These people may not have health records stored elsewhere in the health service so the recording of intervention information with these services is particularly important.

These services may take place in a wide variety of settings in order for them to be accessible to patients. These might include pharmacies, but also community centres, village halls, pubs, places of worship etc. Because of the variety of settings, IT access may not always be possible and pharmacists involved with such initiatives should consider carefully the way in which information might be recorded and stored. These services are likely to take place in an opportunistic way, as directed by the local payor or provider. The unique aspect of these services for pharmacists is that they are not medicines driven.

Home Visits

The pharmacist or member of pharmacy staff visits a patient at their own home for one or more reason. The visit may be because the patient is housebound, but may also be association with a delivery service.

Conclusions

Electronic health records (EHRs) for patients facilitate improved access to patient records for health professionals and patients alike. However, as they contain personal identifiable information, EHRs are subject to stringent confidentiality and information governance requirements and an appropriate consent model and ethical framework of use for EHRs is essential. Due to increased accessability of the patient information on the EHR and the potential for the data to be manipulated for specific purposes or instantiated into other healthcare IT applications, EHRs may be used for improving quality of care and leveraging new services and new ways of working. National care record services may have considerable benefits in providing consistency of patient care and making basic information available to facilitate emergency treatment. However, the relationship of national to local care records is one that requires further research and experience. For all aspects of pharmaceutical care to be supported by EHRs, there is a need to develop a standard format and content for a pharmaceutical care record. This may require considerable work to develop a record structure that supports all aspects of pharmaceutical care in a patient-centred manner and in a way that is consistent with other patient record development initiatives.

References

1. Sjoborg B, Backstrom T, et al. Design and implementation of a point-of-care computerised system for drug therapy in Stockholm metropolitan health region – bridging the gap between knowledge and practice. Int J Med Inform. 2007;76:497–506.
2. For example, the Umbrian regional healthcare system in Italy (see Barbarito F. Regional service card health and social care information system. Presented at opportunities in e-Health, London, 30 Nov 2006).
3. Department of Health. Confidentiality: NHS code of practice. 2003. http://www.dh.gov.uk/en/Publicationsandstatistics/Publications/PublicationsPolicyAndGuidance/DH_4069253. Accessed January 2012.
4. General Pharmaceutical Council. Guidance on patient confidentiality. 2012. http://www.pharmacyregulation.org/sites/default/files/Guidance%20on%20Confidentialiy_April%202012.pdf. Accessed January 2012.
5. General Pharmaceutical Council. Guidance on consent. 2012. http://www.pharmacyregulation.org/sites/default/files/GPHC%20Guidance%20on%20consent.pdf. Accessed January 2012.
6. Pharmaceutical Services Negotiating Committee, Royal Pharmaceutical Society, NHS Employers. NHS information governance: pharmacy contractor workbook. 2010. http://www.psnc.org.uk/data/files/IG/psnc_ig_workbook_2010web.pdf. Accessed January 2012.
7. RCGP Informatics Group. Shared record professional guidance report. 2009. http://www.rcgp.org.uk/pdf/Health_Informatics_SRPG_final_report.pdf. Accessed January 2012.
8. Royal College of Physicians. Developing standards for the structure and content of health records. London. 2008. www.rcplondon.ac.uk/clinical-standards/hiu/medical-records. Accessed January 2012.
9. National Information Governance Board. NHS care records guarantee. http://www.nigb.nhs.uk/guarantee/2009-nhs-crg.pdf. Accessed January 2012.

10. The NHS Constitution. 2010. http://www.nhs.uk/choiceintheNHS/Rightsandpledges/NHSConstitution/Documents/nhs-constitution-interactive-version-march-2010.pdf. Accessed January 2012.
11. Information Commissioner's Office. Subject access to health records by members of the public. 2010. http://www.ico.gov.uk/for_organisations/sector_guides/health.aspx. Accessed January 2012.
12. Royal College of General Practitioners. RCGP records access guide for GPs: sharing records with patients – an evolving process. 2010, v1. http://www.rcgp.org.uk/pdf/Health_Informatics_RecordAccessGPGuide.pdf. Accessed January 2012.
13. Department of Health, Royal College of General Practitioners, British Medical Association. The good practice guidelines for GP electronic patient records. 2011, v4, p. 174. http://www.connectingforhealth.nhs.uk/systemsandservices/infogov/links/gpelec2011.pdf. Accessed January 2012.
14. Shane R. Computerised physician order entry: challenges and opportunities. Am J Health Syst Pharm. 2002;59:286–8.
15. Graez I, Reed M, et al. Care coordination and electronic health records: connecting clinicians. AMIA Annu Symp Proc. 2009;2009:208.
16. Khoury AT. Support of quality and business goals by an ambulatory automated medical record system in Kaiser Permanente of Ohio. Eff Clin Pract. 1998;1:73–82.
17. Marshall PD, Chin HL The effects of an electronic medical record on patient care: clinician attitudes in a large HMO. AMIA Annu Symp Proc. 1998;150–4.
18. Scott RT, Rundall TG, et al. Kaiser Permanente's experience of implementing an electronic medical record: a qualitative study. Br Med J. 2005;331:1313–6.
19. Simonaitis L, Belsito A, et al. Aggregation of pharmacy dispensing data into a unified patient medication history. AMIA Annu Symp Proc. Nov 6, 2008:1135.
20. Smith B. Presented at the guild of Healthcare Pharmacists/United Kingdom clinical pharmacy association Information Technology Interest Group (ITIG) Seminar, Birmingham, Nov 2009. http://www.ghp.org.uk/ContentFiles/ghpitig0911e.pps.
21. Boockvar KS, Livote EE, et al. Electronic health records and adverse drug events after patient transfer. Qual Saf Health Care. 2010;19:e16.
22. Hurdle JF, Weir CR, et al. Critical gaps in the world's largest electronic medical record: ad hoc nursing narratives and invisible adverse drug events. AMIA Annu Symp Proc. 2003;2003:309–12.
23. Smith DH, Perrin N, et al. The impact of prescribing safety alerts for elderly persons in an electronic medical record: an interrupted time series evaluation. Arch Intern Med. 2006;166:1098–104.
24. Orrico KB. Sources and types of discrepancies between electronic medical records and actual outpatient medication use. J Manag Care Pharm. 2008;14:626–31.
25. Mohamed IN, Helms PJ, et al. Using primary care prescribing databases for pharmacovigilance. Br J Clin Pharmacol. 2011;71:244–9.
26. Buck MD, Atreja A, et al. Potentially inappropriate medication prescribing in outpatient practices: prevalence and patient characteristics based on electronic health records. Am J Geriatr Pharmacother. 2009;7:84–92.
27. Roten I, Marty S, et al. Electronic screening of medical records to detect inpatients at risk of drug-related problems. Pharm World Sci. 2010;32:103–7.
28. Berbatis CG, Sunderland VB. Linked electronic medication systems in community pharmacies for preventing pseudoephedrine diversion: a review of internation practice and analysis of results in Australia. Drug Alcohol Rev. 2009;28:586–91.
29. Frenzel JE. Using electronic medical records to teach patient-centered care. Am J Pharm Educ. 2010;74(71).
30. Santana S, Lausen B, et al. Online communications between doctors and patients in Europe: status and perspectives. J Med Internet Res. 2010;12:e20 Accessed January 2012.
31. Montelius E, Astrand B, et al. Individuals appreciate having their medication record on the web: a survey of attitudes to a national pharmacy register. J Med Internet Res. 2008;10:e35.

32. Roblin DW, Houston TK, et al. Disparities in use of a personal health record in a Managed Care Organisation. J Am Med Inform Assoc. 2009;16(5):683–9.
33. Singleton P, Pagliari C, et al. Critical issues for electronic health records: considerations from an expert workshop, Wellcome Trust/Nuffield Trust, London, 2007.
34. Barnet J, Jennings H. Pharmacy information systems in Canada. Stud Health Technol Inform. 2009;143:131–5.
35. Linder JA, Schnipper JL, et al. Electronic health record feedback to improve antibiotic prescribing for acute respiratory infections. Am J Manag Care. 2010;16:e311–9.
36. EC Information Society & Media. The socio-economic impact of intra-operable electronic health record (EHR) and e-prescribing systems in Europe and beyond: final study report. 2009.
37. Brennan N, Mattick K, et al. The map of medicine: a review of evidence for its impact on healthcare. Health Info Libr J. 2011;28:93–100.
38. Smith L, McGowan L, Moss-Barclay C, Wheater J, Knass D, Chrystyn H. An investigation of hospital-generated pharmaceutical care when patients are discharged home from hospital. Br J Clin Pharmacol. 1997;44(2):163–5.
39. Blagburn J, Acomb C. Implementing and evaluating evidence based clinical pharmacy for older people admitted to a secondary care trust. Presented at UKCPA. 2008.
40. Royal Pharmaceutical Society of Great Britain. Guidance on recording interventions. 2006. Available from the Royal Pharmaceutical Society, 1 Lambeth High Street, London, SE7 4JN, UK
41. Schnipper JL, Hamann C, et al. Effect of an electronic medication reconciliation application and process redesign on potential adverse drug events: a cluster randomised trial. Arch Intern Med. 2009;169:771–80.

Chapter 3
Electronic Prescribing and Medicines Administration in Hospitals

Introduction

Electronic prescribing involves the use of computer systems to facilitate the prescription, supply and administration of medicines within a hospital. Electronic prescribing (EP) systems are able to capture a full prescribing history for a patient in a transferrable manner, and open up the potential for use of databases and decision support tools to assist the prescriber in medicine selection. Over the last 10–20 years, EP systems have been developed and used in a number of countries around the world, but their use is by no means widespread.

However, due to sociopolitical developments on a global scale, healthcare providers around the world are increasingly concerned with cost-effectiveness, the increased likelihood of litigation and the need for clinical governance and transparency in healthcare processes. Consequently, there will be an increasing emphasis on the clinical application of information technology to help healthcare providers streamline their business processes and achieve outcome targets. For these reasons, there is an increasing interest in the benefits of EP systems from both healthcare professionals and healthcare provider managers.

Elsewhere in Europe, regional and national healthcare IT programmes have been established to address population healthcare issues [1]. Over the last few years, the Connecting for Health IT programme for the National Health Service (NHS) in England, which ran from 2002 to 2010, has conducted some useful methodology and implementation support work with electronic prescribing in hospitals, but has not designed and delivered a full national solution for electronic prescribing, as first envisaged [2]. Nevertheless, interest in electronic prescribing, in the UK, US and elsewhere, remains high because of the potential benefits that it can deliver, in terms of patient safety and hospital efficiencies.

Since electronic systems for medicine prescribing have been developed independently in different countries, under the auspices of different healthcare systems, it is inevitable that there will be variations in terminology. Furthermore, terms that are not synonymous may be used interchangeably or in an indiscriminate manner.

S. Goundrey-Smith, *Information Technology in Pharmacy*,
DOI 10.1007/978-1-4471-2780-2_3, © Springer-Verlag London 2013

A recent UK definition of electronic prescribing (EP) is as follows:

The utilisation of electronic systems to facilitate and enhance the communication of a prescription or medicine order, aiding the choice, administration and supply of a medicine
through knowledge and decision support, and providing a robust audit trail for the entire
medicines use process

NHS Connecting for Health *Electronic Prescribing in Hospitals: Challenges
and Lessons Learnt* [3].

This is a useful working definition for an EP system because it takes into account
the capacity of an EP system to add value to the patient's prescribing history through
use of clinical decision support tools, and also the process of storage and communication of medicine orders. It is an appropriate description of some of the EP systems
in current use in the UK. It is also a suitable definition for many of the US EP systems that are available at present. However, in the US, electronic prescribing may be
referred to as computerized physician order entry (CPOE), although strictly speak-
ing, this applies to just the prescription data capture process, and not to any decision
support functions, and could be applied to any kind of order (e.g. pathology test etc)
not just a medicine order. Furthermore, the term electronic prescribing is sometimes
incorrectly used to describe the computer generation of a paper prescription (see
Chap. 5), or it may be used to describe electronic transfer of prescriptions (eTP) in
the community, which will be referred to elsewhere in this book.

Benefits of Electronic Prescribing

A review of experience of EP applications in the UK [4] has demonstrated that electronic prescribing implementations have resulted in the following benefits:

- Availability of a fully electronic prescribing history.
- Improvement in legibility and completeness of prescriptions.
- Improvement of hospital business processes due to electronic dissemination of
  prescriptions.
- Availability of electronic decision support tools at the point of prescribing.
- Comprehensive audit trail of prescribing decisions made.
- Reduction in the rate of medication errors.

The benefits of EP systems are far-reaching in significance, in terms of effects on
risk management and risk reduction, and also financial cost. However, it is acknowledged by experts in the field that realisation of these benefits is dependent on system
design, and this will be discussed later in the chapter.

EP systems have particular organisational benefits in the following areas:

1. Reduction of medication errors (including risk reduction in paediatrics, reduction of errors due to barcode medicine administration, and problems associated
   with the increase of errors after implementation in some situations)
2. Workflow management for clinical users of EP systems

3. Discharge Process Efficiency
4. Facilitation of a Seamless Pharmaceutical Supply Chain
5. Reduced use of paper and consumables
6. Clinical System Intraoperability
7. Improvement in hospital business processes due to electronic dissemination of prescriptions
8. Security of prescriptions and prescribing information
9. Quality of care benefits

These benefits will be discussed in the remainder of this chapter.

Reduction in Medication Error Rates with EP Systems

The potential for an electronic prescribing system to reduce medication errors in hospitals is a key benefit of using the system, given the financial cost of medication errors, both in terms of patient morbidity/mortality, cost of care and cost of litigation. For this reason, considerable research has been conducted into the extent to which EP systems can reduce medication errors, particularly in the US, where the practice of medicine is highly litigious.

In US studies, reduction in medication errors following the introduction of EP systems is well-documented. In a key US study from the Brigham and Womens' Hospital, Boston, Mass., Bates et al. [5] compared computerised physician order entry (CPOE), with CPOE plus a team intervention approach, in the prevention of non-intercepted serious medication errors. They found that, with both interventions, during the implementation period, there was a reduction of non-intercepted serious medication errors by 55 %, from 10.7 events per 1,000 patient-days to 4.86 events per 1,000 patient-days (p=0.1). Also, there was a reduction of preventable adverse drug events (ADEs) by 17 % (from 4.69 to 3.88 events per 1,000 patient-days), and a reduction of non-intercepted potential adverse drug events (ADEs) by 84 % (from 5.99 to 0.98 events per 1,000 patient-days). There was found to be no additional benefit of CPOE plus the team intervention over CPOE alone. The error rate reduction figures of 55 and 84 % in this study are substantial, and look impressive, but it must be borne in mind that these figures are for *potential* (non-intercepted) errors, rather than *actual* errors, and it is not clear how many of these potential errors would have become actual errors in practice. The reduction figure for preventable adverse events, 17 %, is considerably smaller.

In a follow-up study, Bates et al. [6] looked at medication errors detected in all patients admitted to three medical wards for a 7–10 week periods in four different years (four points in the implementation process). This study took a broader approach than their previous study, in that it looked across the EP implementation period, and that it looked at the effect of CPOE on all error types, not just serious errors. Data were collected at four points in the implementation period:

(a) Period 1 (1992) – at baseline, before EP implementation.
(b) Period 2 (1993) – EP system implemented
(c) Period 3 (1995) – allergy checking improved
(d) Period 4 (1997) – drug interaction checking and potassium ordering improved

The ADEs were assessed by pharmacists in a structured manner. The study showed that the overall non missed dose medication error rate decreased by 81 %, from 142 ADEs per 1,000 patient-days, to 26.6 ADEs per 1,000 patient-days (p<0.0001). Also, the rate of non-intercepted serious medication errors was reduced by 86 % from baseline to period 3 in the implementation process. However, as discussed, since non-intercepted medication errors are by definition those which are not readily detected under normal circumstances, it is difficult to ascertain whether this reduction was as a result of introducing the EP system. Furthermore, this study also showed that the non missed dose error rate actually increased from period 1 to period 2, despite the overall decrease. The study also showed that the missed dose error rate increased between baseline and period 3, and that the intercepted potential ADE rate increased between the baseline interval and period 2. Again, however, the rise in this latter parameter may not be significant since potential errors may not immediately translate into actual errors.

A US baseline analysis of medication errors [7], involving pharmacist evaluation of 1,111 prescribing errors over a week period, indicated that a significant proportion of these (64.4 %) could be prevented by EP implementation, and that a further proportion (22.4 %) could possibly be prevented, depending on EP system design.

Stone et al. [8] studied error rates with an EP system pre- and post-implementation in an academic surgical unit. They found a very modest level of error reduction; the pre-implementation error rate was 0.22 %, the rate of errors in the first 6 months after implementation was 0.16 %, which rose to 0.21 % after a further 6 months. The fact that this error rate was low and minimally affected by EP implementation may be due to the lack of complex medical regimens in a surgical unit, or because the baseline procedures at the unit were robust. The authors concluded that, while EP systems improved efficiency, they would need to be refined in order to obtain more significant patient safety benefits.

A particular issue with US data on risk reduction with EP systems is the concerning the transcription process. In the US, it is standard practice for hospital staff to produce a drug chart from the physician's clerking notes, and this process is a significant source of medication error in the US setting; some 11 % of errors are as a result of the transcription process. Bates et al. [5] indicated that the rate of non-intercepted errors arising from the transcription process was reduced considerably by 84 %, from 1.3 events/1,000 patient days to 0.2 events/1,000 patient days. Nebeker et al. [9] also commented that the introduction of CPOE, combined with an electronic medication record, had the potential to obviate the need to transcribe orders, and therefore eliminate transcriptions errors. Such a reduction might be expected if an automated system in being used for electronic dissemination of prescriptions to the hospital pharmacy.

Fewer United Kingdom centres have published detailed quantitative studies on risk reductions following EP implementation. Furthermore, it is recognised that, since the healthcare system is different in the UK, the risk profile will be different from the US context. Nevertheless, the incidence of medication errors in the UK has been documented. An analysis of medication errors as part of an assessment of a pharmacy intervention scheme [10], indicated baseline incidence rates of 10.1 % for medicine administration errors, 6.3 % for non-formulary prescribing and 4.6 % for transcription errors. All of these could be reduced by implementation of an EP; again, the transcription error rate could be largely eradicated.

Reductions of errors associated with the prescribing process itself have been noted for some UK EP implementations. Farrar [11] has indicated an increase in the number of complete and correct doses on drug charts, following the introduction of EP. In research information available from the Wirral Trust [12], 2,180 prescriptions for 267 patients were analysed for legibility and completeness, with reference to hospital standards for prescription writing, based on the British National Formulary. Thousand two hundred and seventeen prescriptions generated prior to computerisation and 963 prescriptions generated after computerisation were assessed; electronic prescribing significantly improved the legibility and completeness of prescriptions, compared to prescribing by hand ($p < 0.0001$).

In a review of EP experience at Wirral, presented at the British Pharmaceutical Conference in 1999 [11], Farrar indicated that the use of EP at the Wirral Hospitals had increased the number of complete and correct doses on drug charts from 17.7 % to approaching 100 %. However, the record of medicine administration was not always complete; often once only medicines were completely and correctly prescribed, but no record was made of when they were administered.

In their EP implementation in Ayrshire, Scotland, UK, Fowlie et al. [13] noted a significant reduction in inpatient prescribing errors, and medication administration errors, but a non significant reduction in discharge prescribing errors, following the introduction of an EP system. Their main findings were as follows:

1. The EP system led to a significant reduction in the prescribing error rate for inpatient prescriptions but, interestingly, not for discharge prescriptions. The inpatient prescribing error rate fell from 7.4 % prior to EP implementation, to 7 % 1 month after implementation and then to 4.7 % 12 months after implementation ($p < 0.001$). The decrease in prescribing errors with discharge prescriptions, from 7.5 % prior to implementation, to 5.9 % 12 months after implementation, with an initial increase in error rate to 7.7 % after the first month of EP, did not achieve significance.
2. The EP system led to a significant reduction in medication administration errors, from 9 % prior to implementation, to 6 % 1 month after implementation, and then 5.4 % 12 months after implementation ($p < 0.001$). However, medication administration errors involving intravenous drugs and controlled drugs were omitted from these figures, which could affect the overall medication administration error rate.

The observation that the inpatient prescribing error rate was reduced significantly, but the discharge prescribing error rate was not, may reflect the fact that the discharge prescribing process is innately more structured than the inpatient prescribing process, and therefore the potential for error reduction is greater with the inpatient prescribing process. These authors also showed a significant reduction in medicines administration errors, but indicated that the administration of controlled drugs and intravenous drugs were excluded from this assessment. Inclusion of these groups of medicines, and also implementation of the system in an acute medical area, could both adversely affect the outcome concerning medicines administration errors, due to more complex medicines administration scenarios. Consideration should be given to the design of controlled drug prescribing and administration functions, and also to design of functions for prescribing and administration of continuous infusions and other complex intravenous drug regimens. The latter is particularly complicated, in terms of developing clear user interfaces that support all possible prescribing scenarios, and poor design in this area will lead to the introduction of new errors, resulting in critical incidents.

Shulman and colleagues [14] compared the use of a commercial EP system, without decision support functions, with handwritten prescriptions on an intensive care unit at University College Hospital, London, UK. The study found a moderate reduction of medication errors with the EP system. The medication error rate was 6.7 % (69 errors on 1,036 prescriptions) for handwritten prescriptions and 4.8 % (117 errors on 2,429 prescriptions) for EP generated prescriptions (p < 0.04). In addition, there was evidence that error rates with the EP system decreased gradually following its implementation, due to increasing staff familiarity with the system. When both non-intercepted and intercepted errors were combined, patient outcome scores improved under the EP system. However, the three most serious errors that were identified in this study were with the EP system. While it is clear that EP systems can reduce routine errors, they can lead to facilitation of errors, depending on their design.

Charing Cross Hospital, London, UK, has implemented an commercial EP system (ServeRx, MDG Medical, Israel), which deals with all aspects of medicines management in the hospital environment, including electronic medicines administration, with patient identification using barcode technology, and automated dispensing [15]. The system therefore provides a so-called "closed loop" process, in that it automates all aspects of the medicines management process. The system had a positive effect on both medicine prescribing errors and medicine administration errors. The prescribing error rate fell from 3.8 % (across 2,450 medicine orders) before EP system implementation, to 2 % (across 2,353 orders) after implementation (p < 0.001). Non-intravenous medicine administration errors were reduced from 7 % (across 1,473 non i/v orders) before the implementation, to 4.3 % (across 1,139 orders) after implementation of the system. However, while the system reduced nurse time spent on the medicine administration process, it increased time spent by physicians ordering medicines, and also the time spent by pharmacy staff in providing the ward pharmacy service.

In a study conducted at the Sunderland Hospitals, Beard and Candlish [16] note that current UK hospital drug chart, or "kardex" systems, are probably unacceptable from a risk perspective, and may exceed the UK Health and Safety Executive's threshold of 1 in 10,000 medication errors per year, although there is no specific evidence to show this. The authors indicated that international research had shown

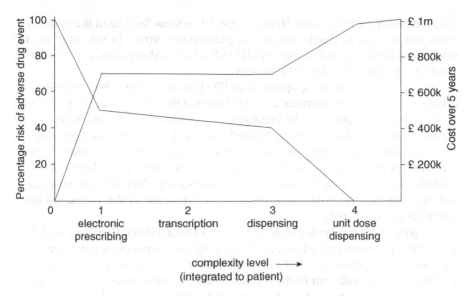

Fig. 3.1 Graph of complexity level of EP system against error reduction and <u>financial cost</u>

that an <u>automated unit-dose drug distribution system</u> was most likely the safest hospital system. On the basis of this research, together with information on error rates at the Sunderland Hospitals, the authors concluded that if such a system were installed at Sunderland, the system was likely to pay for its investment, in terms of harm reduction, within 2–3 years, and that it would be a positive enhancement to <u>clinical governance</u>.

However, the authors noted that, while greater <u>risk reductions</u> could be obtained with systems of increasing complexity, there was a trade-off against the cost of the system. While a unit dose medicines administration system would be the most effective way of reducing <u>error rates</u>, it would be a considerably bigger investment (Fig. 3.1).

However, the problem with this analysis is that, firstly, it does not take into account the proportion of different types of <u>medication errors</u> that might occur in a specific hospital, and, secondly, the way that different systems may introduce new, unrecognised error types, depending on their <u>configuration</u>. This latter issue will be addressed later in this chapter.

However, EP systems do not completely eradicate medication errors. Abdel Qader et al. [17] studied the use of an EP system in a UK hospital in a 4 week retrospective study. They found that, of 7,920 medication orders for 1,038 patients, 664 (8.4 %) were associated with prescribing errors. Omission of drug (31 %), incorrect selection of drug (29.4 %) and dose regimen errors (18.1 %) accounted for most of the errors. Of the 664 errors, 131 (20.8 %) were considered minor, 481 (76.3 %) were considered significant and 18 (2.9 %) were considered serious. The authors concluded that prescribing errors can occur at discharge even with the intervention of an EP system. However, the EP system facilitated the systematic extraction of data to enable analysis of prescribing errors. In this way, the EP system can serve as a tool to identify all kinds of prescribing error, even those that would not be prevented by an EP system.

Quantitative studies on the operation of EP systems have also been published by centres in Europe. Van Doormaal et al. [18] studied the effect of an EP system with clinical decision support on the incidence of medication errors and adverse drug events (ADEs) in a hospital in the Netherlands. They found that the percentage of medication orders containing at least one error dropped from 55 % prior to implementation of the EP system to 17 % post-implementation. While there was also a reduction of ADEs in the hospital after implementation of the EP system, a causal link between the two could not be demonstrated, because of the interrupted time-series design of the study.

In a quantitative evaluation of an EP system in Switzerland, Bonnabry et al. [19] noted that the patient safety benefits of the EP system were dependent on the exact EP functions implemented, and how easy they are for the user to operate. This finding correlates well with Barber's observation that EP systems are not "plug and play" systems, but sociotechnical systems, where the safety of the whole system depends on the interaction of the human operator as well as the operation of the computer [20].

Effect of EP Systems on Medication Error Rates in Paediatrics

Paediatrics is a high risk medical specialty in terms of therapeutics, due to low doses of medicines, complex dosing schedules based on body weight or surface area, drugs being used with a narrow therapeutic index, and non-standard, age related pharmacokinetics of certain drugs. It is likely then that appropriate EP systems could have a beneficial effect on medication error rates in paediatric settings, and a number of studies have been published in this specialty. In a study of paediatric prescribing in five UK hospitals, Ghaleb et al. [21] concluded that EP systems have the potential to reduce dosing errors and errors relating to missing information, but that EP systems would not be rapidly adopted in the paediatric setting. These findings are reflected in the available quantitative studies on paediatric EP at the current time.

Jani et al. [22] studied the use of an EP system in renal patients at a paediatric hospital. The overall error rate was 77.4 % with handwritten prescriptions, which was reduced to 4.8 % following introduction of the EP system. Many of the errors prior to EP implementation were related to important information omitted from the prescription (73.5 %); these errors of omission were most likely reduced by prompts in the EP workflow, when the system was in operation.

Warwick et al. [23] audited prescribing errors and omitted doses before and after EP implementation in a paediatric intensive care unit. They found that the prescribing error rate decreased from 8.8 % prior to implementation to 8.1 % 1 week after implementation (a non significant reduction), and then to 4.6 % 6 months after implementation. Omitted doses were reduced significantly from 8.1 % before implementation, to 1.6 % 6 months after implementation, albeit with a rise to 10.6 % in the week immediately following implementation.

Kazemi et al. [24] studied the error rate for an EP system in a paediatric environment, comparing intervals of physician order entry (POE) and nurse order entry (NOE). They found that prescribing errors decreased from 10.3 % during POE to 4.6 % during the NOE period, and compliance with warnings was 44 % for POE and 68 % with NOE. These results suggest that nurse involvement in the EP process reduced error rates and improved compliance and that, if physicians are resistant to EP implementation, nurse use of the system might facilitate the implementation process.

A US study [25] compared the number of adverse events during 1,200 paediatric hospital admissions, before and after installation of an EP system. Seventy six and ninety four adverse events occurred before implementation, compared to 37 and 35 after implementation, a significant decrease. The system was most effective at reducing adverse events associated with prescribing of aminoglycosides and cephalosporins. The authors concluded that an EP system with comprehensive decision support functions reduced errors associated with paediatric hospital admissions, but that refinements were required to gain further safety benefits.

Jani et al. [26] studied the use of a commercial EP system at a tertiary care children's hospital in the UK. They found that, prior to EP implementation, prescribing errors occurred in 88 of 3,929 items prescribed (2.2 %), and in 57 of 4,784 items prescribed (1.2 %) after implementation. A decrease in the severity rating of errors was also noted after EP implementation. The authors concluded that, while EP appeared to reduce medication errors in the paediatric setting, larger studies were required to assess the impact of EP on error severity, and in different settings.

Current studies suggest that EP has the potential to reduce risks associated with prescribing specifically in a paediatric patient population, in particular errors associated with omission of prescription information. However, as with EP in general patient populations, further studies are required to assess the impact of EP on prescribing errors in detail.

Role of Barcodes in EP Systems

Barcode technology has also been used by EP systems in order to reduce errors in the medication administration process on the ward. The patient's wristband barcode is scanned prior to a medicine administration event to confirm patient identity, and the barcode on the medicine is scanned to confirm the identity of the medicine to be administered. Medicines administration with the assistance of barcodes to identify either the patient or the drug may contribute to reductions in levels of medicine administration errors at the point of administration.

The EP system installed at Charing Cross Hospital, London, UK [15] is a closed loop system, which forced nurses to use the barcode system for patient identification, and it was found that the percentage of patients who were not definitively identified prior to medicines administration decreased from 82.6 % before EP system implementation, to 18.9 % after system implementation.

Poon et al. [27] conducted a study of 115,164 medicines administration events before implementation of barcode medicine administration, and 253,984 administration events after implementation. They found that target adverse events were reduced by 74 % and all adverse events were reduced by 63 %, and that the greater the proportion of doses scanned, the higher the error reduction rates possible. Nolen and Rodes [28] studied the use of barcode medicine administration (BCMA) in anaesthetics for cardiac surgery cases (n = 870). They found that the BCMA process increased the available information on peri-operative drug administration by 21.7 %, and the availability of drug cost data by 18.8 %. Furthermore, the time required to process the operating room anaesthesia record was reduced by 8 min per case, following full implementation of the system.

Miller et al. [29] has indicated that BCMA can reduce medication errors and improve patient safety. However, because the process of medicines administration by barcode scanning is potentially interruptive, there are various work-arounds (BCMA work-arounds) that nurses and pharmacists may use to bypass the system. In a study of five hospitals, Koppel et al. [30] have studied BCMA work-arounds and identified 15 work-arounds, with 31 causes of different types. Reasons for work-arounds [31] include:

• Inability to scan medicines because a scanner is not available at the point of medicines administration
• Lack of awareness of the hospital's BCMA process (bank/agency staff, but also new staff and staff who are not usually involved with medicines administration)
• Shortage of time
• Delay in computer response
• Administration of a medicine prior to prescribing

McNulty et al. [32] discussed strategies for dealing with the problem of BCMA work-around. These include:

(a) encouraging a better culture of ownership of the system among nursing staff
(b) improving the infrastructure to address known technical issues (e.g. wireless black spots)
(c) an effective staff training programme, and better engagement of staff during the implementation period.
(d) greater use of "hard stops" in the system (i.e. ensuring that a medicine is not available for administration without following the procedure – e.g. linking BCMA to ward cabinets). However, hard stops may be highly disruptive and implementers should consider the unintended consequences in each scenario.

The culture of ownership of the system is important and, while BCMA has the potential to resolve many medication errors at the point of administration, managers should remember that different staff groups with have different priorities with BCMA implementation [33]. Pharmacy staff will want to ensure that the stock and inventory is controlled, whereas nursing staff will want to ensure that the system is usable at the point of medicine administration.

The limitations with use of barcodes are the availability, configuration and scalability of appropriate hardware, and also the fact that there are a proportion of medicines that do not have a correct barcode identifier. The use of barcodes may also be limited by harmonisation issues and obsolescence, due to development of RFID (radio frequency identification) technology [34]. In addition, use of barcodes for reduction of medicine administration errors relies on use of original packs (with barcodes) at ward level in a hospital. The use of barcodes in pharmacy professional practice and the pharmacy supply chain will be discussed at greater length in Chap. 7.

Increases in Medication Errors due to the Introduction of EP Systems

An important finding in some US studies is that the implementation of an EP system can actually increase the number of medication errors reported, at least at the outset. In the first of these studies, the Bates 1999 study [6], an increase in error rate was noted during the initial stages of the study, as noted earlier. The increase in error rate was attributed to the EP system's functionality for dealing with potassium orders, which was only finalised later in the implementation process. In the second study, an observational review of a CPOE implementation at the University of North Carolina Hospitals [35], the increase in medication error rate was attributed to (a) increased ability to identify errors due to enhanced data capture on an electronic system, (b) errors generated by staff unfamiliar with a new system, or (c) error detection bias (due to either pre-conceived ideas about EP by users, or evaluators keen to report errors in a new system).

More worryingly, it has been suggested in some studies that the very design of EP systems could facilitate errors, leading to hitherto uncharacterised errors. Koppel et al. [36] did a study of medication errors generated by a commercial EP system that had been in operation in a US hospital for 7 years. They found that the EP system facilitated 22 error types, which fell into two groups: (a) errors generated by the fragmentation of data by the system and lack of integration between the different components of the system, (b) errors arising from the human-machine interface.

Nebeker et al. [9] commented on how a high rate of adverse drug events (ADEs) could occur even at a hospital where there was a high level of IT usage, to support hospital processes. The study looked at ADEs across the electronic prescribing process, by performing a prospective daily review of the electronic medical record for a random sample of all admissions over a 20 week period at a US hospital. The study showed that, of 937 admissions, there were significant ADEs in 483 admissions.

Ninety-nine percent of the ADEs identified resulted in serious harm to the patient, and 27 % of the ADEs were due to medication. The study observed that ADE rates were still relatively high after CPOE introduction, if decision support systems are not present as an integral part of the system. The role of decision support systems in reducing prescribing risk with electronic systems is discussed in detail in the next section.

This phenomenon has also been noted in the UK. As mentioned previously in this chapter, an initial increase in prescribing error rate following implementation of EP (leading to an eventual reduction in error rate), was demonstrated at the Ayrshire and Arran Trust, Scotland [13], for discharge prescriptions, and this observation was responsible for the reduction of prescribing error rate for discharge prescriptions not reaching overall statistical significance. This effect was also noted in the comparative study of an EP system with handwritten prescriptions in the intensive care unit context [14], where the three major errors occurred with the EP system. The authors concluded that clinicians should not become complacent about the use of automated systems to eradicate errors.

A number of subsequent studies have identified the potential for EP systems to generate new errors that would not have occurred prior to use of the system. Flebbe et al. [37] examined the use of an EP system on an orthopaedic surgery ward in a Danish hospital. They found that the EP system could generate new types of error, and that some of these errors could be prevented by improvements in the user interface/workflow, and user training.

Magrabi et al. [38] examined prescribing practice with an EP system in a cohort of hospital doctors under laboratory conditions, to assess the errors that EP system operation could introduce. In the study, 32 doctors completed four tasks, with planned interruptions, and across the four prescribing tasks, an error rate of between 0.5 and 16 % was noted; the wide variation is probably due to the small sample size. A range of different errors occurred in the prescribing process – failure to enter allergy information, incorrect medicine selection, incorrect route, dose, formulation and frequency of administration, and omission of start date, administration times and discontinuation date. Unsurprisingly, complex tasks took longer to complete. The authors indicated that prompts in the workflow may have prevented errors due to task interruption, but that more research was required to evaluate the effects of interruption.

Reckmann et al. [39] conducted a review of 13 hospital EP studies published between 1998 and 2007. While nine of the studies demonstrated a significant reduction in prescribing errors, several studies reported errors such as increased rates of duplicate medicines, and failure to discontinue medicines (although these errors types are possible with paper-based prescribing). The authors concluded that the evidence for the safety benefits of EP systems is not compelling and that further research was required using larger sample sizes, more controlled conditions and standard definitions of errors and adverse events. The issues relating to the methodology of EP study design are discussed in more detail later in this chapter.

Reduction of Medication Errors due to the Availability of Electronic Decision Support Tools at the Point of Prescribing

In the study by Nebeker et al. [9], documenting 937 hospital admissions, it was found that 483 admissions had significant adverse drug events associated with them and that 27 % of these were associated with medication. Of the medication-related adverse drug events, 61 % were associated with prescribing errors and 25 % with monitoring errors and the authors concluded that EP with decision support (DS) features would have a major impact on these error rates, by reducing inappropriate prescribing at the outset, and by providing suitable monitoring tools when certain drugs are prescribed (e.g. digoxin, lithium, theophylline). Indeed, the consensus among electronic pre-scribing specialists is that decision support tools should be an integral part of EP systems, as they have the potential to "add value" to the system as a clinical tool. The above data suggest that DS functions are particularly valuable in reducing selection errors and inappropriate selection at the medicine ordering stage of the medicines management cycle, and thus reduce risks associated with prescribing errors.

Clinical decision support facilities may be classified into active decision support, or passive decision support. Active decision support functions provide a clinical alert to the user automatically as part of the workflow of the system, without the user having to actively seek the clinical information. Active decision support mechanisms are built into the EP system software. Passive decision support functions, however, are stand-alone medicines information reference sources mounted on the internet, an intranet or a local server, and accessible via a "hot key" or quick link by a clinical user, when the user is actively seeking information to resolve a clinical problem.

Clinical decision support warnings and information would include some or all of the following:

(a) sensitivity checking
(b) drug interactions
(c) duplicate therapy/drug doubling
(d) precautions/contraindications
(e) dose checking
(f) formulary status, and
(g) monitoring warnings.

The key issue with active DS functions is that they must be sufficiently comprehensive to be of clinical value, but designed in such a way that they are not excessively presented to the clinical user, which might lead to important warnings being disregarded by the user (warning fatigue). This is a delicate balance and requires considerable thought if the rules are going to be configured within the EP application – for this reason, some implementers have chosen not to support DS functions at all, rather than implement them in a partial manner or without full evaluation; this is the reason why the EP project at Southmead Hospital, Bristol, did not implement any DS functions [40]. In the past, for example, there have been some systems that have limited the number of drug interaction warnings to two or three per drug, or limited the number of allergens for sensitivity checking to two per patient. Limitations of this nature are clearly not acceptable if an EP system is to provide comprehensive DS functions.

However, with a comprehensive DS tool, based on a drug database from a third party data supplier, these issues can be addressed by the mode of implementation of the DS functions in the EP application; with, for example, the use of graded drug interactions, where the system can be configured so that the most clinically significant drug interactions are displayed prominently to clinical users, or flagging of absolute contraindications as a priority. The advantages and disadvantages of using a third party data supplier to enable DS functions will be discussed in the next chapter.

The issue of warning fatigue is well-recognised. On a retrospective analysis of allergy alerts in an EP system, Huntemann et al. [41] found that, out of 49,887 medication orders, 643 orders gave rise to an allergy alert, but that 625 of the 643 alerts (97 %) were overridden, either because the patient had previously tolerated the medication, the benefits outweighed the risk, or for some other reason. The quantitative impact of allergy alerts is therefore low.

Another question to be addressed in the provision of DS is whether there is any type of prescription that should be completely disallowed by a DS function on the EP system – i.e. whether a hard stop should be placed on the prescribing process. There are some prescriptions that are absolutely dangerous and that should (and could) be prevented automatically by an EP system – so-called "never events", for example, intrathecal use of vincristine, daily dosing of methotrexate. The EP system used on the renal unit at the Queen Elizabeth Medical Centre, Birmingham, UK [42] disallowed some orders because of sensitivities and serious drug interactions. However, careful consideration should be given to the issue of disallowing prescriptions because of relative contraindications; if too many prescription types are automatically disallowed, clinicians may choose to bypass the system and write prescriptions by hand, thus defeating the object of an EP system and compromising the completeness of the electronic prescribing record. Strom et al. [43] looked at the use of a hard stop on the co-prescribing of warfarin and co-trimoxazole. They found that, while the alert was highly effective in changing prescribing behaviour (i.e. the prescriber had no choice but to abandon the prescription), it led to clinically significant delays in treatment initiation, which caused the termination of the study.

There are also issues concerning the usefulness of decision support algorithms for alerting on contraindications and high doses. In designing a decision support algorithm for contraindications, Ferner and Coleman [44] remarked that many contraindications were due to co-morbidities, and the decision support algorithm was reliant on relevant clinical data being available in the patient's electronic patient record, which was by no means always the case. Seidling et al. [45] designed an algorithm to alert for high doses of some 170 drugs, taking into account age, renal function and contraindications, but the high dose alert was triggered on only 4.5 % of prescriptions and that clinicians were responsive to only one in four high dose alerts, either because the alert was inappropriate, or the dose prescribed was, in fact, appropriate for the patient. The value of such an algorithm is therefore questionable if its application is limited and it is so readily overridden by the clinician's judgment.

In any case, if systems provide integral application algorithms for calculations (e.g. renal function, hepatic function, body surface area), rather than using a third-party "black box", then clinical users will need to establish whether these are user configurable and how they will be validated and maintained.

Some authors have indicated that use of an EP system made it easier to monitor prescribing habits within a hospital [11]. It is possible to control choice of formulary medicines over non-formulary medicines by the system either (a) guiding prescribers towards formulary medicines, or (b) disallowing prescription of non formulary medicines. Initially, there was some evidence to suggest that EP systems do not have a major impact on the balance of formulary and non-formulary prescribing [46]. However, a number of studies have been published recently suggesting that EP systems can improve therapeutic guideline compliance [47], increase the rate of generic medicine prescribing with a corresponding decrease in branded medicine prescribing [48], and lead to a sustained increase in the rate of generic medicine prescribing, following implementation [49]. All of these effects could lead to a reduction in costs of care by healthcare providers, although the exact costs – and any unintended consequences – will be dependent on the healthcare context.

DS applications have been in use in the US for some years and, due to their potentially pivotal role in preventing medication errors, they have been subject to a great deal of quantitative research in the US medical literature.

Despite some of the potential problems described above, the benefits of DS systems are well-documented. Teich et al. [50] conducted a time series analysis of an EP system where, as new medication orders are entered, the system displayed drug usage guidelines, including dose and frequency information. The EP system led to various positive changes in prescribing practice. These included (a) an increase in the percentage of orders for the formulary recommended drug in a particular drug class; (b) a decrease in the percentage of orders for a drug with doses that exceeded the recommended maximum dose for that drug, and (c) an increase in the use of the approved frequency of administration for a drug.

Hunt et al. [51] performed a systematic review on 68 controlled studies of prescribing DS systems. The effect of a DS system on physician performance was assessed in 65 of the studies and, in 43 of these studies (66 %), a benefit to the physician was demonstrated. A majority of studies demonstrated benefits to the physician for drug dosing systems, preventive care systems and other medical care applications. Physician benefits were not adequately demonstrable for diagnostic DS tools, but the sample size in this review consisted of only five studies. The authors also concluded that further work would be required to assess the impact of DS systems on health outcomes, rather than physician performance.

More recently, there has been a growth in the available literature on specialist applications of decision support and their benefits. The available studies are shown in Table 3.1 below.

Table 3.1 Quantitative decision support studies

Authors	Setting	Decision support intervention	Key findings	Reference
Evans et al.	US hospital	Decision support system for antibiotic prescribing (n=545 patients; control=1,136 patients)	Reduction in number of orders for drugs for which patients had known sensitivities (from 146 orders to 35 (p<0.01)) Reduction of excessive drug doses (from 405 orders to 87 (p<0.01)) Prevention of antibiotic-susceptibility mismatches (reduction from 206 events to 12 (p<0.01)) Reduction in the mean number of days of excessive drug doses (from 5.9 days to 2.7 (p<0.002)) Reduction in the number of adverse drug events caused by antibiotics (from 28 events to 4 (p<0.02))	Evans et al. [52]
Clemens et al.	US hospital	Insulin guideline for non critically ill Type II diabetes patients	The majority of patients did not receive the preferred insulin regimen probably because the guideline was not incorporated into the prescribing workflow in an interruptive manner	Clemens et al. [53]
Bourgeois et al.	US hospital	Acute respiratory infection treatment template	The template reduced inappropriate antibiotic prescribing for acute respiratory infection in children, but overall use of the template was low, again because it was not incorporated into the prescribing workflow in an interruptive manner	Bourgeois et al. [54]
Papaioannou et al.	Canadian Long Term Care Setting	Warfarin monitoring system	Improvement in time to therapeutic range Reduced numbers of INR venepunctures Streamlined prescribing and monitoring processes	Papaioannou et al. [55]
Trafton et al.	US Healthcare Setting	Decision support for opioid prescribing in chronic pain	Use of an iterative process led to development of a multifunctional DS system which was endorsed by clinical guideline authors, content specialists and clinicians	Trafton et al. [56]

Author	Setting	Intervention	Findings	Reference
Milner et al.	US Mental Health Setting	Decision support for prescribing in schizophrenia, bipolar disorder and depression	Increased compliance to mental health treatment guidelines. Providers were adherent for 32 % of their patients in the first 6 months after implementation, and 52 % in the second 6 months	Milner et al. [57]
Tang et al.	Specialist dermatology centre, Singapore	Decision support for isotretinoin prescribing	Increased compliance to isotretinoin prescribing guidance – compliance moved from a baseline of 50–60 % to greater than 90 % for 30 consecutive months post implementation	Tang et al. [58]
Field et al.	US Long Term Medical Setting	Decision support for prescribing in renal patients	Prescribing was more appropriate, and prescribing decisions were of higher quality. Final drug orders were clinically appropriate significantly more often in the intervention group (RR = 1.2 (1.0–1.4))	Field et al. [59]
Lesprit et al.	French Hospital	Decision support system prompting post-prescrition review of antibiotic prescriptions	Reduced number of days of antibiotic therapy in the intervention group (p<0.0001). Improved quality of antibiotic prescribing. Greater compliance to the recommendations of the attending physician	Lesprit et al. [60]
Buising et al.	Australian Hospital	Computerised antimicrobial approval system	Appropriate increase in prescriptions for broad spectrum antibiotics. Corresponding reduction in third and fourth generation cephalosporins, carbapenems etc. Improved susceptibility of Pseudomonas spp to many antibiotics. No increases in adverse outcomes for patients with Gram negative bacteraemia	Buising et al. [61]
Cooley	US Hospital	Venous thromboembolism (VTE) risk calculator	The system reduced the incidence of VTE by 41 %. In 2008, 2,050 alerts led to a pharmacist intervention, of which 85 % were accepted by medical staff. However, with only 33 % of the alerts was prophylaxis actually prescribed	Cooley [62]

In the US, the Joint Clinical Decision Support Workgroup (JCDSWG) has published recommendations for EP system DS function development [63]. The group recognised that the benefits of DS functions used in EP systems had not been fully realised, and that further development of DS systems was required. They reported recommendations and action plans in three general domains:

- advances in system capabilities (DS knowledge base, database elements, usability and performance).
- standardisation and centralisation of vocabularies and knowledge structures, so that standard DS routines do not need to be adapted by software vendors and healthcare providers.
- financial and legal incentives to promote adoption of DS within EP systems.

However, research by Wang et al. [64] has shown that, on average, available EP systems in the US fulfill only half of these recommendations. It is this lack of advanced functionality that will need to be addressed before EP systems can have a positive effect on financial cost and health outcomes in chronic diseases in the US; this is one of the issues addressed by the Medicare Modernisation Act 2003. In response to these publications, Miller et al. [65], highlighted the ability of large academic medical centres to implement complex EP systems, but that smaller, rural healthcare providers do not have the expertise or financial resources to implement such system. Furthermore, Miller et al. claimed that, while the DS functions of well-established EP systems at centres of excellence are often maintained in house, the third party drug database used in commercial EP systems that would be implemented elsewhere may not be of such high quality. Miller and colleagues argue for the development of US-wide drug database and terminology standards to support DS, and indicated that EP systems would not be implemented widely across the US, in rural areas as well as major conurbations, until that happened.

Problems with Evaluating Risk Reduction Aspects of EP Systems

With many of the quantitative studies described here, whose purpose is to perform a statistical analysis on error rates and other risk issues in the medicines management process, and to evaluate an EP system as an intervention in the process, there are potential confounding factors. These may include the following:

(a) the subjectivity of reviewers in the evaluation of adverse drug events and medication errors in these studies;
(b) the lack of parallel studies between units with EP and those without EP in the same hospital;

(c) the extent to which the study period represents the full implementation schedule of the EP system. If certain functions of an EP system are not available, this may have a profound effect on the error rates detected by a quantitative study.

(d) error detection bias in error reporting, due to the vigilance of researchers and users when evaluating a new system, and

(e) the extent to which the benefits reported are specific to the working practices of the sites studied.

The extent to which these confounding factors associated with research methodology or system design affect benefits needs to be evaluated in more detail.

A number of papers have commented on the methodology of quantitative evaluations of EP systems. In a systematic review, Ammenwerth et al. [66] noted that, while EP systems can reduce the risk of medication errors, quantitative studies varied considerably in their setting, design, quality and results. The authors called for more randomized controlled trial methodology covering a wider range of clinical settings and geographical locations. Similarly, following their review of EP studies, Reckmann et al. [39] called for greater control of EP study conditions, larger sample sizes and standardized definitions of error types.

It has been suggested [67] that there should be a formal methodology for validation of EP software, analogous to the process of licensing a new medicine. However, while a prospective, controlled study is the "gold standard" in clinical medicine, and especially therapeutics, to demonstrate associations and causal links, such studies are much harder to design to assess clinical informatics interventions.

In his discussion of the methodologies for evaluation of EP systems, Trent Rosenbloom [68] describes a number of problems in the design of clinical informatics studies, including (a) the isolations of specific system variables to be tested, (b) the choice of the most appropriate units of study (individual patient, ward, consultant list or hospital) to be exposed to the system variable under study conditions, and (c) ensuring that the study groups remain distinct during the time that systems or workflows are tested, and that there is no inadvertent cross-over of subjects.

While there is a clear need for quantitative data on the operation of EP systems, the insights that qualitative techniques can provide should not be discounted. Savage et al. [69] compared medication error rate pictures obtained by quantitative and qualitative methods at an English hospital after implementation of an EP system. They concluded that, while the two processes provided an similar picture of the drug use process, interviews took less time to conduct than retrospective record review (and were therefore more cost-effective), provided more information on the prescribing process, identified two errors that were not found in record review and provided reasons for delayed or omitted administration of medicines.

Barber et al. [20] reviewed progress with implementation of EP systems, evaluating the implementations at Burton on Trent, and Charing Cross Hospital, London, in the UK. They concluded that, although EP systems reduce medication errors, their implementation is not straightforward, and they should always be regarded as work in progress. Effectiveness of EP systems should be regularly monitored, because of changing human systems and test platforms. Green [70] has commented on the perception in health services that EP systems can eradicate medication errors and reduce the need for clinical pharmacists. The likely situation however is that, given the need for ongoing monitoring of EP systems for effectiveness and emergence of new errors, the need for clinical pharmacy input is likely to remain, if not increase, in order to achieve the lowest possible medication error rates within a hospital.

Workflow Management for Clinical Users of EP Systems

Clinical professionals of all disciplines face a two-fold task in their daily practice in a healthcare environment. On the one hand, they have a duty of care towards their patients, and an obligation to ensure that patients are treated in a way that fulfils legal requirements and ethical requirements, and most closely represents accepted best practice for their profession. On the other hand, there are operational pressures from the healthcare organisation to treat patients as quickly and efficiently as possible and to achieve statistical benchmarks and service level targets. Furthermore, these two objectives can sometimes seem to be in opposition; best care of the patient by the practitioner may be at the expense of meeting organisational targets. However, there is a greater chance of both objectives being achieved if workflow for the practitioner – both the prescriber of a medicine and the person administering the medicine – is streamlined by the appropriate use of electronic systems.

For many healthcare systems, designed for use in a busy working environment, the design of the user interface is important. For an application such as electronic prescribing, where there is a need to present complex prescribing information in a way that enables appropriate professional decision making, and to input comprehensive medicine order information in a straightforward and timely manner, user interface design is critical. An appropriate user interface is one of the key factors contributing to the reduction of medication errors by EP systems.

The obvious benefit of EP system is a legible and complete prescription, facilitated by the electronic display of that information. Thus, an EP system can ensure that, for every prescription, the following details will be included:

- Medicine
- Form/Formulation
- Strength
- Dose
- Route
- Frequency
- Duration (if applicable)
- Any specific prescribing or administration instructions

The legibility and completeness of prescriptions is beneficial to the working practices of all system users involved in the prescribing, dispensing and administration of medicines. Two UK implementations of EP systems have commented on the positive impact of EP on the legibility and completeness of the prescribing record

[12, 40]. The legibility and completeness of an electronic prescription are dependent on other factors.

Firstly, the legibility of prescription information on an electronic system in the clinical environment cannot be assumed; it will depend on (a) the design of the screens and forms used to display the data, (b) fonts and styles of text used, (c) graphics and colours used on the screens. The adoption of chart designs and form templates that were already in use in the hospital, as happened in Burton on Trent, UK [71], will facilitate staff familiarization with the system and, as well as having a positive effect on the reduction of prescribing errors and medicine administration errors, will increase staff confidence in the system and the efficiency with which the EP system is used.

Secondly, the completeness of the displayed prescribing history will depend on the completeness of the prescription data captured in the first place. To facilitate adequate prescribing data capture, the database structure should have sufficient granularity, and the medicines data should be sufficiently comprehensive to handle a wide range of complex prescribing scenarios. This is because, in general terms, many prescriptions generated in secondary care are more complex and varied than those in primary care.

For example, a secondary care EP system would need to include:

(a) a comprehensive range of routes (including routes to support enteral feeding)
(b) a comprehensive range of formulation types,
(c) reducing/increasing dose regimens (e.g. prednisolone reducing dose),
(d) loading doses and associated maintenance doses of the same drug (e.g. gentamicin),
(e) alternate routes of administration for the same drug dose (e.g. metoclopramide 10 mg po/pr/im),
(f) complex administration instructions (e.g. co-trimoxazole 960 mg on Monday, Wednesday and Friday). The provision of adequate functionality to allow capture of complex drug orders is important because, in two reports [11, 72], it was found that errors of omission increased after EP implementation, because prescribers found themselves unable to enter certain types of prescription due to the design of the system and the configuration of the drug data.

Other issues associated with data capture concern the use of screen prompts and the use of freetext fields. Firstly, it has been demonstrated that functions to prompt the user to fill in each line of the form in the prescribing workflow help to minimize missing information and maximize patient safety [73]. Secondly, in an analysis of 2,914 electronic prescriptions with free text fields, it was found that there were internal data discrepancies in 16.1 % of prescriptions, leading to adverse events in 83.8 % of cases and severe adverse events in 16.8 % of cases [74]. Many of the discrepancies were between structured and free text fields, and the study authors indicated that designers should use free text fields with care in the prescribing workflow.

In addition to the clear display of a prescribing history for a patient, another important issue in facilitating an efficient workflow for the user is the ease of operation of the system. For any EP system, there is a balance between the completeness of data capture during the prescribing process, and ease and usability of the system for the prescriber. A system might have a 12 stage prescribing process to enable the clinician to prescribe a complex regimen, but this may not be acceptable a busy clinician using the system. One way of addressing this issue might be to use pre-defined orders (PDOs) for commonly used prescriptions (e.g. Furosemide 40 mg Tablets – one to be taken each morning), so that the clinician can select a complete medication order in a single process. This approach was used in a pilot at Southmead Hospital, Bristol, UK [40] to speed up the prescribing process and to incorporate implicit decision support, in the form of prescribing guidance. However, use of PDOs may lead to different kinds of error due to incorrect selection of a PDO, or errors within a PDO being propagated inadvertently through large numbers of patient records.

As well as the number of operations required to generate an electronic medicine order, in terms of defining the order details – medicine, form, strength, dose, route, frequency etc – consideration needs to be given to the number of confirmation boxes ("double dares") and warning messages that appear during the workflow for different types of prescribing. It is well recognised that, if a system presents an excessive number of clinical warnings in any particular workflow, especially warnings that are irrelevant to the specific prescribing scenario, the user will begin to ignore the warnings (so-called "warning fatigue").

The need for confirmation boxes may be reduced by the appropriate use of control default options and highlighting, but the risk management implications of these developments need to be considered carefully. Furthermore, due to the increasing granularity of data – both coded data from patient records, and drug data within decision support systems – decision support data providers are now looking at aggregated querying techniques to produce single warning messages that are more intuitive to the particular prescribing scenario.

Just as the prescribing workflow of an EP system can affect the efficiency with which clinicians prescribe medicine, so the medicine administration workflow of an EP system can streamline the process of medicines administration in a hospital environment. As with the prescribing workflow, the medicine administration workflow is highly dependent on the user interface and the screen layout.

The medicines administration workflow must have appropriate forms and controls to present the administration of various different medication types that might be administered in hospitals, such as:

- Regular medicines – those given at regular intervals (e.g. amlodipine 10 mg daily)
- When required (PRN) medicines – those given when necessary (e.g. paracetamol for pain relief, also antiemetics post surgery)
- Once only (stat.) medicines (premedication for surgery or vaccines)
- Fluids (e.g. 0.9 % sodium chloride, or 5 % dextrose)
- Continuous infusions

In order to present the complexities of all prescription types in a concise manner, some EP systems have chosen to design a medicines administration screen that, to a greater or lesser extent, mimics the traditional medicine chart or Kardex, with sections for each of the prescription types – regular, when required, once only, fluid and

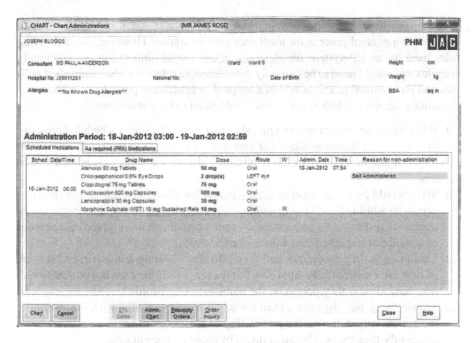

Fig. 3.2 Layout of an EP system medicines administration screen (by kind permission of JAC Computer Services Ltd)

continuous infusions. Figure 3.2 shows the design of a medicines administration screen for scheduled (regular) medicines on an EP system. This allows administration of the medicine within a defined timeframe, and also provides other functions to support medicines administration (witnessing for CDs, referential data on the medicine etc).

In an EP system, the design of the administration screen will facilitate and manage the medicines administration process. For example, the different order types might be displayed on different tabs on screen, so that the nurse can view all active orders according to order type. Scheduled orders – due at a particular time – could be displayed distinctively – for example, highlighted in red. The order could then revert to the standard background once the administration had been recorded (or alternatively show in, for example, green for a set period of time after the administration had been recorded, to indicate that it was a current administration that had recently been done). For regular medicines, there would be a facility to input a user code for the person administering the medicine; for other order types, there should be a facility to record a user code, a date and time of administration and a dose, where a variable dose is required. With all scheduled order types, there should be the facility to record a missed-dose code.

Alternatively, all of the orders scheduled to be given at any given time could be displayed on one administration screen, regardless of order type. The disadvantage of this, however, is that they may not be immediately viewable alongside the whole record of prescribed medication.

Electronic medicine administration has the advantage that it can force users to conform to a general process for medicines administration. However, the underlying rules used by an EP system for electronic medicine administration are potentially complex and would need to be carefully considered, in relation to the established policies and professional practices within a hospital or healthcare provider organisation.

Among others, the following issues would need to be considered:

(a) What would be an appropriate time window for highlighting a scheduled prescription as due for administration? For example, with a regular medicine, the system might highlight it in red for an hour either side of the scheduled administration time

(b) What would be an appropriate time window for allowing a scheduled prescription to be administered? For example, with a regular medicine, the system might enable recording of an administration (cells active and highlighted) for an hour either side of the scheduled administration time.

(c) Should once only medicines and fluids display as being administrable as soon as they are electronically signed by the prescriber? If they are not administered, how long should they persist on the administration profile?

(d) Should "lock out" functions exist for when required medicines?. For example, the system might disable the prescribing of paracetamol based analgesics more frequently than every 4 h and at doses of more than eight tablets in 24 h.

Other issues that would need to be considered in detail would be the design of administration functions for continuous infusions and controlled drugs, the configuration of missed dose codes and the provision of an on-hold and off-hold facility for items that have been prescribed, but which need to be withheld pending other events, for example pathology test results. The latter function is useful in a number of situations involving elective treatments – for example chemotherapy.

Discharge Process Efficiency

One of the most beneficial features of an implementation of EP at Salford, UK [75] was the introduction of immediate discharge summaries (IDS). These were piloted in medical and care of the elderly wards in mid 2001, and rolled out to the whole hospital in 2002. This function enabled clinicians to assemble an electronic discharge summary for each patient, including drug ordering from picklists or pre-defined orders.

The rationale for the IDS function was to streamline the hospital discharge process, which is a significant issue in the UK context. If the process for patient discharge is inefficient then not only is quality of care reduced and patient/healthcare professional morale affected, but bed management in the hospital becomes difficult, and this has far-reaching implications for service planning and development. Another significant issue with the hospital discharge process is that, with the traditional consultant's letter, it takes some time for a patient's care plan – and current medication schedule – to be sent to the patient's GP. The quadruplicate discharge forms introduced recently have been a considerable improvement, but these can be – and often are – mislaid by patients and hospital staff. Electronic communication of hospital discharge information from secondary care to primary care constitutes a critical factor in addressing some of the logistical and communication issues associated with a patient's discharge from hospital.

In recent years, while UK hospitals have been waiting for a national EP solution from NHS Connecting for Health, many UK hospitals have sought to develop interim electronic solutions for managing the discharge process, therefore addressing a key issue for many hospitals. Some of these solutions have been implemented in a standalone fashion, others as a conscious step towards a full EP solution.

Two examples of UK electronic discharge systems are the eDischarge system at the Southampton Hospitals, UK, and the electronic transfer of care system at the Princess of Wales Hospital, Bridgend, Wales, UK. At Southampton [76], an e-discharge module was implemented as part of the Ascribe pharmacy management system. The system was piloted in the acute medical unit (AMU) in 2007. Based on this pilot, a second version of the software was launched on the medicine and care of the elderly wards and subsequently rolled out across the Trust. The system provides a direct transfer of discharge information to 30–40 GP surgeries in the locality, and a range of clinical and financial audit functions for hospital users. At the Princess of Wales Hospital, Bridgend [77], an electronic transfer of care system was developed in house to ensure that electronic information on a patient's medicines and care plan was generated and distributed to GPs in a timely manner. The system enabled discharge information to be available to primary care clinicians on the day of discharge for 96 % of patients, a considerable improvement on previous paper-based systems.

Kirby et al. [78] conducted a case–control study of 102 patients processed by the electronic discharge system installed at King's Mill Hospital, Derbyshire, UK. They found a dramatic reduction in the time taken to process a hospital discharge with the electronic system, in comparison with the traditional paper-based discharge process (from a mean time of 80 days, to a mean time of 0 days (p < 0.0001)).

Work has also been done on the development of a common electronic discharge tool for hospitals throughout Wales, UK, using the Welsh Clinical Portal [79]. The system provides a common drug database and dose syntax (to support communication of prescribed doses) based on the dm+d medicines terminology. At the time of writing (early 2012), this system is about to be piloted in Cardiff and Vale Health Board.

Facilitation of a Seamless Pharmaceutical Supply Chain

Many of the inefficiencies of existing manual prescribing and medicine supply processes in hospitals surround the way in which prescriptions written on the wards are filled with actual medicines from the hospital pharmacy department. Consequently, a direct link between each ward and the pharmacy department, either as different workstations in a networked EP system, or as an interface between an EP hub and a pharmacy system, represents the means for automating order transfer between wards and the pharmacy, and a valuable tool for reducing inefficiency in the pharmacy requisition process.

In addition to the way that an EP system can streamline medicine ordering and supply within a hospital, it has been suggested that EP systems can help to facilitate a seamless pharmaceutical supply chain from manufacturer to patient. For over 20 years, hospital pharmacists in many countries have been using departmental pharmacy systems for procurement and stock control of medicines. More recently, automated dispensing systems (pharmacy robots) have been introduced to increase the accuracy of the dispensing process. Furthermore, with the availability of web-based intranets and the associated security technology, together with the growth of e-commerce and the regulatory framework to support it, many pharmaceutical wholesalers are looking to promote e-procurement of medicines by hospitals. Moreover, many hospital pharmacies are seeking to implement e-procurement, with the stock movement and control efficiencies that it can provide.

Consequently, there now exists the means for a seamless pharmaceutical supply chain from the pharmaceutical industry to pharmaceutical wholesalers, and then via central procurement agencies and hospital pharmacies to the patient.

To this end, the baseline specification for the English Connecting for Health electronic prescribing programme proposed a number of functionalities that were intended to streamline the medicines supply chain. These included:

(a) an electronic link from the ward to the pharmacy for placing orders
(b) interface with hospital pharmacy systems
(c) automatic escalations for overdue medicines
(d) support for newer stock control methodologies such as 28-day dispensing and patient's own drugs (PODs),
(e) supply chain tracking in real time (viewable by patient), and
(f) medicine costs to be displayed throughout the supply chain.

While many of these requirements may seem straightforward, there are various implications of providing these functions. Firstly, as many implementers have already found out, the interface of an EP system to an (existing) pharmacy system may not be straightforward, in terms of interface building and data configuration. Furthermore, provision of price information for medicines is problematic, both in terms of appropriate adjustments for actual and notional costs, and maintaining the data in real time, throughout the system, at each point of the supply chain. Secondly, supply chain tracking which includes the wholesaler would require involvement of wholesaler systems staff to provide a link between hospital EP systems and NHS e-procurement processes, and the complexities that would involve. Thirdly, provision of supply chain information to patients, as the end-user, would potentially increase the number of disputes between the pharmacy department and wards concerning throughput issues.

It is highly desirable that an EP system should support the various stock control methodologies currently used in hospital pharmacy – 28 day dispensing, use of patients' own drugs (PODs) etc. These will be discussed in greater detail in Chap. 6. However, as with clinical pharmacy tools, this represents an area that is unique to hospital pharmacy, and pharmacy managers should have an active role in the design of these functions.

Reduced Use of Paper and Consumables

Traditionally, hospital records have been used and stored in a paper format. As well as the clinical notes pages, the records include pro forma results pages for radiology and other departmental investigations and mount sheets for pathology result slips. The records for one patient will have different sections in the clinical notes for each specialty and admission, together with outpatient appointments. As a consequence, the records for a patient who has had a long history of chronic disease and/or multiple acute referrals to clinicians of different specialties may fill several folders and occupy up to 50 cm of shelf-space in A4 format. The difficulties associated with the storage and retrieval of such records have driven the developments in patient administration systems (PAS) and clinical coding over the last 30 years. Specifically, hospital inpatient prescribing records have been recorded on a medicine chart, or Kardex. During any one admission, a patient may have a number of different charts, some of which might be overflow charts with only one or two entries on, prior to the aggregation of the patient's current prescriptions on a single new chart. Multiple drug charts leads to the risk of inadvertent medicine duplication, where a medicine is prescribed in error on more than one chart.

The introduction of electronic prescribing and medicine administration will therefore reduce the amount of consumables used by a health provider – charts, paper, pens etc. Depending on the size of the healthcare provider, the resulting savings may be significant. Nevertheless, while these savings may represent a clear, unambiguous and relatively easily measurable benefit of introducing an EP system, they are insignificant compared to the costs of wasted staff time due to inefficient paper-based systems and processes, and the possible costs of litigation when errors are made, as a result of these inadequate processes. However, unlike savings on paper and consumables, costs for staff time and potential litigation are more difficult to calculate, and it will be tempting for health providers not to attempt to quantify them.

Clinical System Intraoperability

The ability of different clinical systems to interact with each other in an integrated manner is a key factor in the streamlining of healthcare business processes within a hospital or healthcare provider. This is especially the case given the disparate nature of many business processes within a healthcare enterprise, and the silo development of individual departmental systems in the past.

In a number of UK EP implementations, authors have commented on the ability of an EP system to provide a complete and comprehensive prescribing history, which is interfaced with the hospital electronic health record (EHR) system [40, 71, 80]. This reduces the number of lost or absent medication records, facilitates remote electronic prescribing and enables the easy production of hard copy discharge prescriptions and other supporting information from different locations. A US study has shown that, where an EP system is integrated with an EHR system (in line with the meaningful use requirements), the physician is more likely to consult the patient's prescribing history than when EP is provided as a stand-alone system [81].

With EP system interfaces or integration, there is therefore the potential for transferability of the prescribing history to and from other systems. For example, this enables electronic prescriptions to be routed to the hospital pharmacy departmental system, to streamline the medicine supply process, as discussed previously. This would also enable pathology test orders to be triggered from within the EP system, and sent to the pathology system, and for pathology test results to be posted to the EP system.

As mentioned previously, a comprehensive prescribing history within an EP system is important for ensuring evidence-based working practices and user confidence in the system. However, when the system is designed to provide an optimally comprehensive prescribing record, there are complications associated with the actual transfer of high-granularity prescription data between systems. While transfer of data may be relatively uncomplicated within a system in a physical or wireless networked environment, or through interfaces with other systems in the same hospital location, there are issues associated with transferring data to external systems. There is, for example, currently no model in the UK for transferring medicines data from hospital EP systems – where they exist – directly to GP systems or community pharmacy systems in primary care.

This is a key driver for regional or national healthcare IT programmes, where prescription information is transferred to a central spine, from which it may be retrieved by other healthcare providers as the need arises. Apart from technical issues concerning architecture and hardware, standards for interoperability are required for data formats and messaging. With healthcare application data entities and structures, the international messaging standards are the Health Level 7 (HL7) formats, which are based on XML conventions. For data relating to medicines, the standard terminology is SNOMED CT, from which comes the terms for the UK dictionary of medicines and devices (dm±d) [82]. However, at the present time, there is still work to be done on the definition of messages to allow transfer of prescription information between systems at the level of complexity required to support secondary care EP, and also on the ability of applications to receive these messages.

Improvement in Hospital Business Processes due to Electronic Dissemination of Prescriptions

As mentioned previously, clinical practice in healthcare provider organisations is undertaken in the context of a health economy and practitioners are under pressure to achieve health outcome targets and service level agreements. These pressures exist irrespective of whether the health economy is insurance-driven, as in the US and many countries in continental Europe, or based on central government funding, as with the UK National Health Service. Consequently, healthcare managers in any context are receptive to the use of electronic systems to facilitate greater efficiencies in the use of healthcare resources in a provider organisation.

A number of studies have postulated organisational efficiencies as benefits of using an EP system. However, more than perhaps any other EP system benefit area, organisational benefits cited for EP systems are most dependent on the political and socioeconomic contexts in which they are demonstrated. For example, one US study, which reviewed the design of EP software, concluded that detailed system design was important to clinical users and determined how rapidly systems were adopted [83]. The authors concluded that EP design required continuous assessment to ensure relevance to routine practice and user acceptability. This conclusion is consistent with the observation with UK implementations that EP is a "sociotechnical system" and needs to be constantly monitored and developed to deal with unintended consequences of system use in routine healthcare practice [20].

Furthermore, organisational benefits of EP systems are also dependent on the structure and objectives of the study in which they were demonstrated.

Organisational efficiency benefits cited in studies include:

(a) reduced medication ordering turn-around times.
(b) reduced hospital stay times,
(c) streamlining of the hospital discharge process (an important issue in the UK context),
(d) reduced pathology test and radiology test reporting times
(e) reduced number of pathology orders generated, and
(f) improved patient record documentation.

Some studies have indicated that EP has a beneficial effect on medication ordering turnaround times, which is not surprising as many systems facilitate the seamless transmission of prescription data from a prescribing workstation on the ward to a pharmacy system in the pharmacy. One US study has identified a 64 % average reduction in medication ordering turn-around time following implementation of an EP system [35]. Another US study [84] looked at the effect of EP systems compared to paper prescribing on dose compliance with first doses of antibiotics. This study found that, with the EP system, there was greater compliance with antibiotic orders, and the medication was delivered to the patient significantly faster than with paper prescribing. A third US study has suggested that EP systems can have a positive effect on the total hospital stay time [5], but this is harder to demonstrate conclusively and may not be replicated in the UK context.

Nevertheless, two of the UK reports indicate that EP is a useful tool for the clinical pharmacist, and helps to streamline the pharmacist's work in terms of the prescription review process, thus allowing them to spend more time on near-patient clinical activities [71, 80].

One important factor in the streamlining of hospital prescribing processes is the ability of the electronic prescribing record to be viewed remotely in a number of different locations.

Security of Prescriptions and Prescribing Information

As discussed in Chap. 2, the requirement for confidentiality on the part of health-care professionals is well-established in legislation and in professional standards. The growth of electronic records in healthcare, together with the increased likelihood of electronic dissemination of electronic patient information in local, regional or even national systems beyond the provider institutions has caused health professionals and providers alike to become more concerned about the confidentiality of electronic patient records. The information governance agenda covers a range of issues relating to information management and security, and IG requirements will cover the following:

• Appropriate use of passwords or Smartcard technology for log in
• Data transfer and encryption
• Security of hardware devices and premises where equipment is used
• Training on confidentiality and management of IG incidents

There are many features in hospital EP systems, which deliver IG and information security requirements. Systems will have password protection, and role-based access, so that users will only have access to the functions of the system that are appropriate to their role. Hospital EP systems will be mounted on dedicated servers and networks, so may be regarded as a closed system, and therefore more secure than traditional paper charts, which are liable to being lost or viewed by unauthorized users.

There are, however, some potential areas of concern. Firstly, the security of wireless networks in different clinical areas should be scrutinized. Secondly, depending on the architecture of the system in terms of the number and type of workstations on each ward, there may be specific training requirements for users concerning system security (for both hardware and software access) and data protection. As a rule, the need for information security should be weighed up against the hazards posed by system security arrangements that are too stringent. A simple example of this is that, if the system log on procedure is too complex, users may be tempted to remain logged on at their usual workstation, than to log off between users, which may be counterproductive to information security.

A hospital implementing EP will need to determine how the database of users, their roles and access permissions can be maintained, given the fact that there is often an extensive and high-turnover pool of users (locums, bank staff etc), and that role-based access is an important deliverable for interoperable systems, which is a goal for implementers where there is a regional or national healthcare IT programme.

Quality of Care Benefits

The reduction of medication errors and improvement in the quality of prescribing are now well-documented benefits of EP systems. The use of the PICS EP system at Birmingham University Hospitals, UK, [85] had a positive impact on quality of care, due to enforcement of local clinical guidance and policies. This included:

- Implementation of the Trust antibiotics policy
- Daily alert if a patient's prescription does not follow the venous thromboembolism risk assessment guidelines.
- Automatic switching to generic statins for cost reduction, where appropriate.
- Automatic prescribing of methicillin-resistant Staph. Aureus (MRSA) decolonization medication in patients found to be MRSA positive.

However, there is still little information on whether EP systems have a positive impact on actual patient outcomes, as a result of their influence on clinical practice. One study, by Michelis et al. [86], looked at whether EP use could improve goal attainment in low density lipoprotein (LDL) levels in patients with hyperlipidaemia in an outpatient setting. Prescribing records were reviewed retrospectively for an EP system which did not use decision support for hyperlipidaemia guideline adherence, but did include formulary decision support, which gave clinicians information about drug costs. Patients receiving electronic prescriptions were 59 % more likely to achieve their LDL goal than patients who received paper prescriptions. The authors suggested that this may be because patients whose prescriptions were generated electronically were more likely to receive a generic statin, and this would have a positive impact on optimum dosing.

Further research is required on the impact of EP on actual clinical outcomes, as opposed to healthcare outcomes targets, for various therapeutic areas and public health issues. Nevertheless, there may be difficulties in controlling studies in such a way that a clear causal effect can be seen on a clinical outcome as a result of using an EP system, rather than due to other clinical or environmental factors.

Conclusion

There is considerable research to show that electronic prescribing (EP) and medicines administration systems have the potential to reduce the number of medication errors and improve patient safety in hospitals. They also have possible benefits in improving the medicines use workflow in hospitals and may have benefits in improving care outcomes. However, it is also recognized that EP systems can introduce new kinds of medication error, depending on their design and implementation. For this reason, implementers should monitor systems carefully during the post-implementation phase to identify any unintended clinical consequences of the use of the system. The most important aspect of EP systems, where they can add value to the prescribing process in hospitals, is the availability of electronic decision support tools as part of the prescribing workflow. EP systems should be regarded as "sociotechnical systems" in that their safe and effective use is not only dependent on the EP software, but on the hospital procedures and human operators that surround the software. This is especially the case with barcode medicine administration, where users can and will find work-arounds to the system. There is a need to consider how EP systems can be integrated into a wider medicines management IT architecture in hospitals, with links to community systems.

References

1. For example, the Umbrian regional healthcare system in Italy (see Barbarito F. Regional service card health and social care information system. In: Presented at opportunities in e-Health, London, 30 Nov 2006) and the Stockholm Regional Drug Prescribing System in Sweden (See Sjoborg B, Backstrom T, et al. Design and implementation of a point-of-care computerised system for drug therapy in Stockholm metropolitan health region – bridging the gap between knowledge and practice. Int J Med Inform 2007;76:497–506).
2. Gandecha R, Klecun E, et al. What the National IT Programme means for pharmacy and pharmacists. Pharm J. 2005;275:56–60.
3. NHS Connecting for Health. Electronic prescribing in hospitals: challenges and lessons learnt. 2009. p. 9. http://www.connectingforhealth.nhs.uk/systemsandservices/eprescribing. Accessed April 2012.
4. Goundrey-Smith SJ. Electronic prescribing – experience in the UK and system design issues. Pharm J. 2006;277:485–9.
5. Bates DW, Leape L, et al. Effect of computerised physician order entry and a team intervention on prevention of serious medication errors. J Am Med Assoc. 1998;280:1311–6.
6. Bates DW, Teich JM, et al. The impact of computerised physician order entry on medication error prevention. J Am Med Inform Assoc. 1999;6:313–21.
7. Bobb A, Gleason K, et al. The epidemiology of prescribing errors: the potential impact of computerised physician order entry. Arch Intern Med. 2004;164:785–92.
8. Stone WM, Smith BE, Shaft JD, Nelson RD, Money SR. Impact of a computerised physician order entry system. J Am Coll Surg. 2009;208:960–7.
9. Nebeker J, Hoffman JM, et al. High rates of adverse drug events in a highly computerised hospital. Arch Intern Med. 2005;165:1111–6.
10. Dodd C. Assessing pharmacy interventions at Salisbury Healthcare NHS Trust. Hosp Pharm. 2003;10:451–6.
11. Farrar K. Accountability, prescribing and hospital pharmacy in an electronic, automated age. Pharm J. 1999;263:496–501.
12. Farrar K. In: Smith J, editor. Building a safer NHS for patients: improving medication safety. London: Department of Health; 2004.
13. Fowlie F, Bennie M, et al. Evaluation of an electronic prescribing and administration system in a British Hospital. Pharm J. 2000;265(Suppl):R16.
14. Shulman R, Singer M, et al. Medication errors: a prospective cohort study of handwritten and computerised physician order entry in the intensive care unit. Crit Care. 2005;9:R516–21.
15. Franklin BD, O'Grady K, et al. The impact of a closed-loop electronic prescribing and administration system on prescribing errors, administration errors and staff time: a before and after study. Qual Saf Health Care. 2007;16:279–84.
16. Beard R, Candlish C. Does electronic prescribing contribute to clinical governance? Br J Healthc Comput. 2004;21:27–9.
17. Abdel Qader DH, Harper L, Cantrill JA, Tully MP. Pharmacists' interventions in prescribing errors at hospital discharge: an observational study in the context of an electronic prescribing system in a UK teaching hospital. Drug Saf. 2010;33:1027–44.

18. Van Doormaal JE, van den Bemt PM, et al. The influence that electronic prescribing has on medication errors and preventable adverse drug events: an interrupted time-series study. J Am Med Inform Assoc. 2009;16:816–25.
19. Bonnabry P, Despont-Gros C, et al. A risk analysis method to evaluate the impact of a computerised provider order entry system on patient safety. J Am Med Inform Assoc. 2008;15:453–60.
20. Barber N. Electronic prescribing – safer, faster, better? J Health Serv Res Policy. 2010;15 Suppl 1:64–7.
21. Ghaleb MA, Barber N, et al. The incidence and nature of prescribing and medication administration errors in paediatric inpatients. Arch Dis Child. 2010;95:113–8.
22. Jani YH, Ghaleb MA, et al. Electronic prescribing reduced prescribing errors in a pediatric renal outpatient clinic. J Pediatr. 2008;152:214–8.
23. Warrick C, Naik H, Avis S, Fletcher P, Franklin BD, Inwald D. A clinical information system reduced medication errors in paediatric intensive care. Intensive Care Med. 2011;37:691–4.
24. Kazemi A, Fors UG, Tofighi S, Tessma M, Ellenius J. Physician order entry or nurse order entry? Comparison of two implementation strategies for computerised order entry system aimed at reducing dosing medication errors. J Med Internet Res. 2010;12:e5.
25. Holdsworth MT, Fichtl RE, et al. Impact of computerized prescriber order entry on the incidence of adverse drug events in pediatric inpatients. Pediatrics. 2007;120:1058–66.
26. Jani YH, Barber N, Wong IC. Paediatric dosing errors before and after electronic prescribing. Qual Saf Health Care. 2010;19:337–40.
27. Poon EG, Cina JL, et al. Medication dispensing errors and potential adverse drug events before and after implementing bar code technology in the pharmacy. Ann Intern Med. 2006;145:426–34.
28. Nolen AL, Rodes 2nd WD. Bar-code medication administration system for anesthetics: effects on documentation and billing. Am J Health Syst Pharm. 2008;65:655–9.
29. Miller DF, Fortier CR, et al. Barcode medication administration technology: characterisation of high-alert medication triggers and clinician workarounds. Ann Pharmacother. 2011;Feb:epub.
30. Koppel R, Wetterneck T, et al. Workarounds to barcode medication administration systems: their occurrences, causes and threats to patient safety. J Am Med Inform Assoc. 2008;15:408–23.
31. Van Onzenoort HA, Van den Plas A, et al. Factors influencing bar-code verification by nurses during medication administration in a Dutch Hospital. Am J Health Syst Pharm. 2008;65:644–8.
32. McNulty J, Donelly E, et al. Methodologies for sustaining barcode medication administration compliance. A multi-disciplinary approach. J Healthc Inf Manag. 2009;23:30–3.
33. Agrawal A, Glasser AR. Barcode medication. Administration implementation in an acute care hospital and lessons learned. J Healthc Inf Manag. 2009;23(4):24–9.
34. Adcock H. European association of hospital pharmacy congress: RFID raises issues associated with privacy and data collision. Hosp Pharm. 2006;13:138.
35. Spencer DC, Leininger A, et al. Effect of a computerised prescriber order entry system on reported medication errors. Am J Health Syst Pharm. 2005;62:416–9.
36. Koppel R, Metlay JD, et al. Role of computerised physician order entry systems in faciliating medical errors. J Am Med Assoc. 2005;293:1197–203.
37. Flebbe E, Jensen T, Andersen P. Does electronic medicine prescription cause new types of errors? Ugeskr Laeger. 2009;171:2260–4.
38. Magrabi F, Li SY, Day RO, Coiera E. Errors and electronic prescribing; a controlled laboratory study to examine task complexity and interruption effects. J Am Med Inform Assoc. 2010;17:575–83.
39. Reckmann MH, Westbrook JI, Koh Y, Lo C, Day RO. Does computerised provider order entry reduce prescribing errors for hospital inpatients? A systematic review. J Am Med Inform Assoc. 2009;16:613–23.
40. Gray S, Smith J. Practice report – electronic prescribing in Bristol. Healthc Pharm. 2004;(August):20–2.
41. Hunteman L, Ward L, et al. Analysis of allergy alerts within a computerised prescriber order entry system. Am J Health Syst Pharm. 2009;66:373–7.

42. Nightingale PG, Adu D, Richards NT, Peters M. Implementation of rules-based computerised bedside prescribing and administration: intervention study. Br Med J. 2000;320:750–3.
43. Strom BL, Schinnar R, Aberra F, Bilker W, Hennessy S, Leonard CE, Pifer E. Unintended effects of a computerised physician order entry nearly hard stop alert to prevent a drug interaction. Arch Intern Med. 2010;170:1578–83.
44. Ferner RE, Coleman JJ. An algorithm for integrating contraindications into electronic prescribing decision support. Drug Saf. 2010;33:1089–96.
45. Seidling HM, Schmitt SP, Bruckner T, Kaltschmidt J, Pruszydlo MG, Senger C, Bertsche T, Walter-Sack I, Haefeli WE. Patient specific electronic decision support reduces prescription of excessive doses. Qual Saf Health Care. 2010;19:e15.
46. Ross SM, Papshev D, Murphy EL, Sternberg DJ, Taylor J, Barg R. Effects of electronic prescribing on formulary compliance and generic drug utilisation in the ambulatory care setting: a retrospective analysis of administrative claims data. J Manag Care Pharm. 2005;11:418–9.
47. Went K, Antoniewicz P, et al. Reducing prescribing errors: can a well-designed electronic system help? J Eval Clin Pract. 2010;16:556–9.
48. Fischer MA, Vogeli C, et al. Effect of electronic prescribing with formulary decision support on medication use and cost. Arch Intern Med. 2008;168:2433–9.
49. Stenner SP, Chen Q, Johnson KB. Impact of generic substitution decision support on electronic prescribing behaviour. J Am Med Inform Assoc. 2010;17:681–8.
50. Teich JM, et al. Effects of computerised physician order entry on prescribing practices. Arch Intern Med. 2000;160(18):2741–7.
51. Hunt DL, Haynes B, Hanna SE, Smith K. Effects of computer-based clinical decision support systems on physician perfomance and patient outcomes: a systematic review. J Am Med Assoc. 1998;280(15):1339–46.
52. Evans RS, Pestotnik SL, Classen DC. A computer-assisted management program for antibiotics and other antiinfective agents. N Engl J Med. 1998;338:232–8.
53. Clemens E, Cutler T, et al. Prescriber non-compliance with a new computerised insulin guideline for non critically ill adults. Ann Pharmacother. 2011;Jan:18.
54. Bourgeois FC, Linder J, et al. Impact of a computerized template on antibiotic prescribing for acute respiratory infections in children and adolescents. Clin Pediatr (Phila). 2010;49:976–83.
55. Papaioannou A, Kennedy CC, et al. A team-based approach to warfarin management in long-term care: a feasability study of the MEDeINR electronic decision support system. BMC Geriatr. 2010;10:38.
56. Trafton JA, Martins SB, et al. Designing an automated clinical decision support system to match clinical practice guidelines for opioid therapy for chronic pain. Implement Sci. 2010;5:26.
57. Milner KK, Healy D, et al. State mental health policy: implementation of computerized medication prescribing algorithms in a community mental health system. Psychiatr Serv. 2009;60:1010–2.
58. Tang MB, Tan ES, et al. Australas J Dermatol. 2009;50:107–12.
59. Field TS, Rochon P, et al. Computerized clinical decision support during medication ordering for long-term care residents with renal insufficiency. J Am Med Inform Assoc. 2009;16:480–5.
60. Lesprit P, Duong T, et al. Impact of a computer-generated alert system prompting review of antibiotic use in hospitals. J Antimicrob Chemother. 2009;63:1058–63.
61. Buising KL, Thursky KA, et al. Electronic antibiotic stewardship—reduced consumption of broad-spectrum antibiotics using a computerized antimicrobial approval system in a hospital setting. J Antimicrob Chemother. 2008;62:608–16.
62. Cooley T. Presented at the guild of healthcare pharmacists & UK clinical pharmacy association joint conference 2009. Clin Pharm. 2009;1:291.
63. Teich JM, Osheroff JA, Pifer EA, the CDS Expert Review Panel. Clinical decision support in electronic prescribing: recommendations and an action plan. J Am Med Inform Assoc. 2005;12:365–76.

64. Wang CJ, Marken RS, Meili RC, et al. Functional characteristics of electronic prescribing systems: a field study. J Am Med Inform Assoc. 2005;12:346–56.
65. Miller RA, Gardner RM, Johnson KB, Hripcsak G. Clinical decision support and electronic prescribing systems: a time for responsible thought and action. J Am Med Inform Assoc. 2005;12:403–9.
66. Ammenwerth E, Schnell-Inderst P, et al. The effect of electronic prescribing on medication errors and adverse drug events: a systematic review. J Am Med Inform Assoc. 2008;15:585–600.
67. Summers V. Association of Scottish chief pharmacists. Electronic prescribing – the way forward. Pharm J. 2000;265:834.
68. Trent Rosenbloom S. Approaches to evaluating electronic prescribing. J Am Med Inform Assoc. 2006;13:399–401.
69. Savage I, Cornford T, Klecun E, Barber N, Clifford S, Franklin BD. Medication errors with electronic prescribing (EP): two views of the same picture. BMC Health Serv Res. 2010;10:135.
70. Green C. Look to the future and see the opportunities. Clin Pharm. 2011;3:34.
71. Curtis C, Ford NG. Paperless electronic prescribing in a district general hospital. Pharm J. 1997;259:734–5.
72. Fowlie F, Bennie M, Jardine G, Bicknell S, Toner D, Caldwell M. Evaluation of an electronic prescribing and administration system in a British Hospital. Pharm J. 2000;265(Suppl): R16.
73. Connor AJ, Hutton P, Severn P, Masri I. Electronic prescribing and prescription design in ophthalmic practice. Eur J Ophthalmol. 2011;21:644–8.
74. Palchuk MB, Fang EA, et al. An unintended consequence of electronic prescriptions: prevalence and impact of internal discrepancies. J Am Med Inform Assoc. 2010;17:472–6.
75. Clark C. Information technology in action. Hosp Pharm. 2002;9:109–12.
76. Pepperrell M, Patel N. Presented at the guild of Healthcare Pharmacists/United Kingdom Clinical Pharmacy Association Information Technology Interest Group (ITIG) seminar, Birmingham, Oct 2010. E-Discharge Summary. http://www.ghp.org.uk/ContentFiles/ghpitig10e.pps.
77. Lewis R. Presented at the guild of Healthcare Pharmacists/United Kingdom Clinical Pharmacy Association Information Technology Interest Group (ITIG) seminar, Birmingham, Nov 2009. "What's wrong with a piece of paper?" The Electronic Transfer of Care. http://www.ghp.org. uk/ContentFiles/ghpitig0911e.pps.
78. Kirby J, Barker B, et al. A prospective case control study of the benefits of electronic discharge summaries. J Telemed Telecare. 2006;12(S1):20–1.
79. Rose D. Presented at the guild of Healthcare Pharmacists/United Kingdom Clinical Pharmacy Association Information Technology Interest Group (ITIG) seminar, Birmingham, Oct 2011. E-Discharge with Formulary Control. http://www.ghp.org.uk/ContentFiles/ghpitig11e.pps.
80. Foot R, Taylor L. Electronic prescribing and patient records – getting the balance right. Pharm J. 2005;274:210–2.
81. Desroches CM, Agarwal R, Angst CM, Fischer MA. Differences between integrated and stand-alone E-prescribing systems have implications for future use. Health Aff. 2010; 29:2268–77.
82. Frosdick P, Dalton C. What is the dm + d and what will it mean for you and pharmacy practice? Pharm J. 2004;273:199–200.
83. Khajouei R, Jaspers MW. The impact of CPOE medication systems' design aspects on usability, workflow and medication orders: a systematic review. Methods Inf Med. 2010;49:3–19.
84. Cunningham TR, Geller ES, Clarke SW. Impact of electronic prescribing in a hospital setting: a process-focused evaluation. Int J Med Inform. 2008;77:546–54.
85. Slee A. E-prescribing in Birmingham. In: Presented at the guild of Healthcare Pharmacists/ United Kingdom Clinical Pharmacy Association Information Technology Interest Group (ITIG) seminar, Birmingham, Oct 2010. http://www.ghp.org.uk/ContentFiles/ghpitig10a.pps.
86. Michelis KC, Hassouna B, et al. Effect of electronic prescription on attainment of cholesterol goals. Clin Cardiol. 2011;34:254–60.

Chapter 4
Pharmacy Automation

The use of robots and other automated devices to pick and pack items were developed to support the logistics and retail industries and have been commonplace in these sectors for many years. However, the uptake of these technologies to support pharmacy services has been a fairly recent development. The drivers for this have been increasing dispensing workloads over the last 20 years, the need to achieve cost-efficiencies in the health service and an increased emphasis on patient safety in recent years.

Pharmacy robots have been used in some US hospitals from the mid-1990s, where the use of unit-dose dispensing, and a need to charge each unit to a cost centre in an insurance based health service, is more conducive to the use of robots. However, robots were not widely adopted in UK hospitals until some years later.

In the UK in 2001, the Audit Commission's report, A Spoonful of Sugar [1], looked at medicines management in hospitals, advocated the "re-engineering" of pharmacy processes to improve efficiency and particularly highlighted the potential for pharmacy automation to reduce dispensing errors and to free up staff time for near-patient clinical activities. This led to a rapid adoption of robotics in UK hospital pharmacies in the early years of the twenty first century. However, pharmacy robots have been less extensively adopted in community pharmacy (especially in the UK), although they offer some of the same benefits. This situation may change, however, with the emergence of community pharmacies with higher prescription throughput, the increasing emphasis on patient-focused pharmacy services and the adoption of unit dose robots to handle residential homes dispensing.

The use of automation at ward level – for example, automated dispensing cabinets – can not only reduce medicine administration errors, but also support changes in traditional pharmacy working practice. Ward automation has not as yet been widely adopted in the UK, but is an area of considerable potential.

Remote dispensing, using remotely-operated kiosk units, has the potential to extend the availability of a pharmacy service – both in terms of timing and location – as well as ensuring an accurate dispensing process. However, the use of these devices is limited in the UK at the present time due to the legislation surrounding the supervision of pharmacies. In addition, there are various automated solutions to handle specific aspects of the dispensing process – for example, the dispensing of methadone mixture (methadone dispensing) to registered drug misusers.

This chapter explores the various technologies which are in use to automate the pharmacy dispensing and medicine supply process, describes their benefits and some of the key problem areas, and highlights areas for potential future development.

History and Development of Dispensary Technology

Over the years, pharmacists have used various technological innovations to automate and streamline the medicine dispensing process. The development of electronic tablet counters in the 1970s enabled pharmacy staff to dispense large quantities of routinely-used tablets; such devices, based on optical light-beam technology, became commonplace during the 1980s. The introduction of pharmacy computer systems (pharmacy systems) in the 1980s for labeling and stock control had a profound impact on the operational and strategic management of hospital pharmacies. The functionality of these will be discussed in full in a later chapter, but the arrival of pharmacy systems were responsible for automating the medicine labeling process, which was very laborious when done with a typewriter.

In continental Europe and the United States where, in many cases, there are insurance-based healthcare systems, the dispensing of medicines developed on an original pack basis. The first automated dispensing systems, or pharmacy robots, designed for original packs, were developed for use in hospitals and healthcare facilities in Europe and America, and there is considerable experience of their implementation in these parts of the world [2].

Patient pack and unit dose dispensing facilitates the use of automated systems for the storage, stock management, picking and labeling of medicines because:

(a) the need for bulk dispensing of loose tablets and capsules is eliminated
(b) an automated system can control stock on a pack by pack, or dose by dose, basis rather than having to maintain a complex database of pack details for every medicinal product

In the past, automated dispensing systems were not widely adopted in the UK in the same way as in the US because UK hospitals have traditionally had a mixed dispensing profile, with some bulk dispensing, especially of high-volume medicines (e.g. paracetamol, co-codamol 8/500), together with the use of manufacturer's original packs (of varying quantities) for other formulations.

However, since the European Community Directive 92/97 became law in 1999, there has been a gradual move towards original pack dispensing in the UK, which has been encouraged by various UK stakeholders. The adoption of original pack dispensing in the UK has facilitated consistency in prescribing and pack quantities, and this has made automated dispensing systems a viable possibility in UK hospital pharmacies.

Pharmacy Robot Design and Operation

There are various manufacturers of <u>pharmacy robots</u> in both the US and Europe. In the US, there are many suppliers, the best known of which are Kirby Lester, who pioneered tablet-counting technology in the 1980's, and McKesson, a large healthcare IT provider. In Europe, pharmacy robots are supplied by ARX Ltd, Mach4 Pharma Systems, Robopharma, Willach and a number of other suppliers.

ARX is the market leader in the UK with, at the time of writing, 631 installations across 350 sites in the UK, including a large number of NHS hospitals. Mach 4 Pharma Systems Ltd (formerly Wesfalia Systems) have 23 operational sites in the UK NHS, including the Royal Brompton Hospital and the East Cheshire Hospital at Macclesfield.

Robopharma have implementations at Whiston Hospital, Merseyside, and in community pharmacies in the UK. Willach Pharmacy Solutions have installed robots into a number of UK community pharmacies.

In addition, there are two systems that have been installed in UK sites, but are no longer on the market for future installations. The Swisslog Packpicker has been installed at two hospital sites – Charing Cross Hospital, London, and Royal Liverpool and Broadgreen. The Baxter Consis system has five installations – at New Cross Hospital, Woiverhampton, the Oxford Radcliffe Hospitals Trust, Dartford Hospital (two installations) and Bedford Hospital.

The technical operation of pharmacy robots has been reviewed in detail by Swanson [3]. The ARX Rowa Speedcase, the ARX flagship product which was installed in many UK hospitals, has a <u>picking head</u> situated on a track between two parallel sets of vertical shelving. The Speedcase may be installed as a single unit, but many hospitals opted for tandem installation in order to increase picking speed, and so that one picking head can provide backup if the other fails. ARX developed fridge and controlled drugs storage units for the Speedcase, in order to increase the proportion of dispensary stock that can be stored by the robot. The performance of the Rowa <u>cold storage units</u> have been independently validated [4]. Storage of stock in the system is on a random storage basis, where the operating software assigns to the stock to a random location within the device. The software controls the movement of stock within the machine, alternating between picking, which is given priority, and putting stock away, which is done when the dispensing workload is low. The earlier implementations of the Speedcase required manual and semi-automated loading of stock, where the barcode (GTIN Code/European Article Number (EAN)) (<u>EAN code</u>) of each pack is scanned, and then pack dimensions are measured, to verify pack identification and to assign it to shelf space, before the items are placed on an input conveyor belt. Rowa subsequently produced an automatic loading module (the Pro-Logic, or Pro-log) [5]; items are emptied into a hopper, and the loading process can take place while the device is unattended. It can therefore be run overnight. Rowa also offer combined random access and channel modalities and <u>multiple pack supply functionality</u> (Flash-pack), but, while these increase supply capacity, they are at the expense of in-line labeling. Rowa has also developed the Robodose system, a pouch-based <u>unit dose dispensing system</u>, which may in future provide a solution to monitored dosage system (MDS) based dispensing. The latest ARX robot is the Vmax, which has a V-shaped picking head allows for multiple pack picking and therefore greater efficiency. As with other robot types, Vmax units can be used together. Up to nine packs at a time can be moved on the picking head, and each unit can pick up to 2,400 packs per hour.

Mach 4 Pharma Systems produce two automated dispensing systems – the Medimat system and the Speedbox system. The Medimat system, which operates in a similar way to the Speedcase, with random storage and semi-automatic loading, is suitable for low to medium turnover dispensing. It can be installed as a multiple unit, the Multi-Medimat. The Speedbox system is more suitable for dispensing high-turnover items and is a channel device. Mach 4 provides a solution whereby both systems can be installed as an integrated unit, to deal with a range of dispensing throughput. In this scenario, the Medimat provides a semi-automatic load for both it and the Speedbox unit, but the two devices operate independently as far as picking is concerned. Mach 4 also market an automatic loading unit, the Fill-In Box, and a unit-dose device, the Unidose.

The Swisslog Packpicker is in common use in Europe, and but has only two installations at UK hospitals [3], and is not actively marketed in the UK. The Packpicker consists of two or more storage modules consisting of a honeycomb design, with different cell sizes to cater for different sized packs. The system can therefore deal with a wide range of pack sizes. Like the Speedcase, storage in the device is on a random storage basis, and the loading process is semi-automatic, with the barcode and product dimensions being scanned, prior to the product being assigned shelf space.

The operation of the Baxter Consis system is significantly different to the Speedcase and Packpicker. Product storage in the Consis is on a channel storage basis, rather than a random storage basis. The stock is loaded manually into prede-termined, gravity-fed channels. The picking head selects a pack from the lower end of each channel. A Consis may have a single picking head, or a multiple picking head, or a combination of the two modalities. The advantage of the Consis, with its channel storage system, over the earlier random storage devices is that it offered a far higher storage density (around 3,300 packs/m^2), with a relatively small floor area (footprint). The Consis also has software to perform an accuracy check at the end of the dispensing process, checking the picked product against the label generated by the pharmacy system.

Adoption of Pharmacy Automation in the UK

The pharmacy of St Thomas' Hospital, London, installed an ARX ROWA Speedcase device in 2000 [6]. At the time, only 150–200 products were stored in the robot. A significant number of products could not be dispensed by the robot – for example, controlled drugs, fridge items (CD and refrigerated storage units for the Speedcase were not available at that time), unlicensed medicines and bulky or fragile items. However, installation of the device reduced the amount of storage space required in the dispensary, and freed up space for a counselling area, to enable the pharmacy team to provide a more patient-focussed service.

Another early adopter of pharmacy automation was the Wirral Hospitals NHS Trust [7]. In 1999, the Wirral Hospital formulated a business case for the introduction of an automated dispensing device, with the projected benefits being (a) redeployment of pharmacy staff to the wards, and (b) possible reduction in dispensing errors. The Wirral Hospitals chose an ARX Rowa Speedcase, and the system went live in 2001. The system held 8,000 items (80 % of the dispensary stock) and had an interface with the JAC pharmacy system. At this point, the system still had manual loading, and labeling of items was still a manual process.

In 2003, a number of hospitals installed automated dispensing systems. The Royal Wolverhampton Hospital became the first UK site to install a Baxter Consis system [8]. The system was set up with two picking heads – one for single items and one for multiple items – with a total of 11,000 items stored in the device. At the time of go-live, controlled drugs could not be stored in the Consis system.

The Royal Liverpool and Broadgreen Hospitals installed a Swisslog Packpicker [3], with five picking heads and labelling stations, handling 1,200 high usage product lines. However, at that point, the system could not accommodate CDs, fridge items or bottles larger than 300 ml. The installation of the robot enabled the pharmacy dispensing process to be redesigned to support clinical services.

In 2003, ARX Rowa Speedcase machines were also installed at the Whittington Hospital [9] and the Royal Free Hospital [10], and a Swisslog Packpicker was installed at Charing Cross Hospital [3] Also, at that time, the first automated dispensing device to be installed in Wales was installed at the West Wales Hospital, Camarthen [11] – again, a tandem configuration Speedcase. The device was used for dispensing and ward box filling; furthermore it has the capacity to provide remote out of hours supplies by on call pharmacists, an important benefit in a rural area.

Robots have also been used to enable off-site centralized medicine supply. NHS Greater Glasgow and Clyde installed pharmacy robots at their regional pharmacy distribution centre, which replaced 14 pharmacy stores in the Glasgow area [12]. This enables centralized medicine supply to hospital wards and direct to homecare patients. The centre holds 12 day's pharmacy stock, totaling £2 m in value, and distributes to 4,500 destinations per week. 96 % of items are delivered correctly first time. Supply problems and medicine shortages account for the other 4 %, although there may be occasional operator errors with the robots. The robotic distribution centre has enabled pharmacy staff to be redeployed in ward-based clinical pharmacy teams.

Table 4.1 shows details of published references to UK implementations of pharmacy robots in hospitals.

Robots have also been implemented in a number of community pharmacies in the UK, mainly to support a high dispensing throughput and enable the pharmacy to develop patient-focused services.

Table 4.1 Published references to UK Hospital pharmacy robot implementations

Hospital	Device	Reference
St Thomas' Hospital, London	ROWA Speedcase	Gross [6]
Wirral Hospitals	ROWA Speedcase	Slee et al. [7]
New Cross Hospital, Wolverhampton	Baxter Consis	Fitzpatrick et al. [8]
Royal Liverpool and Broadgreen Hospital	Swisslog Packpicker	Clark [13]
Whittington Hospital, London	ROWA Speedcase	Coleman [9]
Royal Free Hospital, London	ROWA Speedcase	Anon [10]
West Wales Hospital, Camarthen	ROWA Speedcase	Anon [11]
NHS Greater Glasgow and Clyde	ROWA	Taheri [12]

Figure 4.1 shows a typical implementation of a pharmacy robot in a local acute hospital.

Drivers for Use of Automation in Pharmacy

As mentioned previously, the Audit Commission's report "A Spoonful of Sugar: Medicines Management in UK Hospitals" [1], published in 2001, highlighted the importance of both original pack dispensing and the use of pharmacy automation to improve patient safety and release pharmacy staff to perform patient-centred pharmacy services. This was a key stimulus for adoption of pharmacy robots in the UK. Following on from the publication of this report, many hospitals in the UK developed a business case for, procured and implemented an automated dispensing system, or pharmacy robot, for their dispensaries.

Another key driver for pharmacy automation has been the application of Lean methodology [14] to streamline the processes of the entire organization within a hospital or healthcare provider. Lean was developed by Toyota production engineers and has been adapted widely in the automotive industry and now in the construction, retail and healthcare sectors. The Lean method is a way of reviewing and improving work systems to enhance the processes that are fundamental (value) and eliminate waste (non-value), to arrive at the optimum way of working, which is accepted by the culture of the whole organization. The Lean method was used in the reorganization of pharmacy work processes at Bolton Hospital UK.

There have been a number of national quality drivers in the England NHS which have been a major stimulus to the installation and use of pharmacy automation. These include the CQUIN (Commissioning for Quality and Innovation) framework and the QIPP (Quality, Innovation, Productivity and Prevention) programme [15]. Automation meets requirements for these initiatives by being innovative technology which prevents dispensing errors, improves efficiency of the dispensing process (both in terms of throughput and use of space) and thereby has a positive effect on quality of care (patient waiting times and redeployment of staff on near patient pharmacy services).

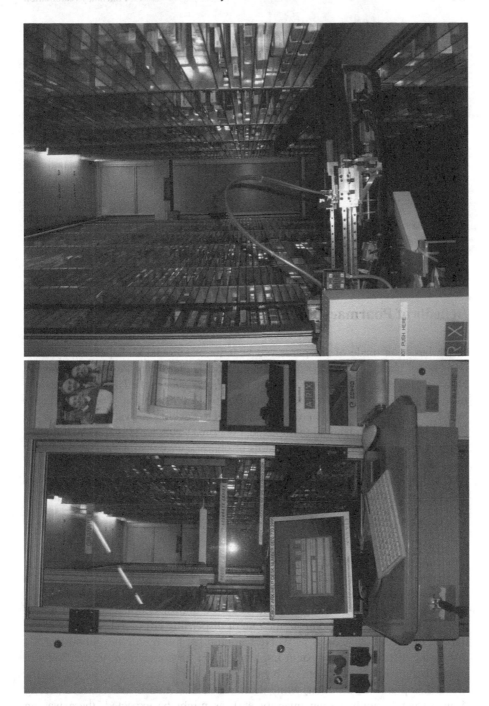

Fig. 4.1 Dispensary robot at Gloucester Hospital, UK

In addition, a number of larger community pharmacies in the UK have adopted pharmacy robots to streamline the dispensing volume, and to enable them to deliver other pharmacy services, such as medicines use reviews (MURs) and other clinically focused services, which rely on the availability of a pharmacist for consultation.

The theoretical and perceived benefits of automation are:

(a) a reduction in dispensing errors;
(b) rationalisation of the dispensing process, leading to efficiencies in dispensary throughput and turnaround times, and
(c) re-engineering of pharmacy services, which might include the development of a ward-based medicines management service, and decentralisation of the clinical pharmacy service.

However, there are few published papers which quantify the actual benefits of pharmacy robots. The evidence-base for pharmacy robots benefits is discussed in the next section.

Benefits of Pharmacy Robots

Much has been made of the perceived benefits of automated dispensing systems (benefits of pharmacy robots) in policy documents and the professional literature. However, in the early stages of adoption of these devices in the UK, there was very little quantitative evidence for these benefits [16]. For this reason, researchers at the Welsh School of Pharmacy were commissioned to develop an evaluation toolkit for those sites that were planning to implement pharmacy robots. This section discusses the published information on the benefits of pharmacy robots for dispensing.

A number of implementers have published data on the benefits that they have realised on implementing an automated dispensing system. There are three main areas where pharmacy automation has contributed to development of best practice:

• Reduction in Dispensing Errors

The Wirral Trust [7] found that, in the 4-month period after implementation of their Speedcase, the rate of dispensing errors had been reduced by 50 %. This is consistent with the fact that, in previous dispensing error logs, the most common dispensing errors at the Wirral were incorrect product selection, and incorrect product strength selection – both of which would be almost eliminated by the use of pharmacy automation. In contrast, the rate of dispensing errors following the introduction of the Baxter Consis at Wolverhampton [8] fell by a more modest 16 %, during the 4 months after system implementation, in comparison to the 5 month period before implementation. A breakdown of the dispensing error results for Wolverhampton indicates that, while there was a reduction in other errors (wrong drug, wrong strength, wrong quantity etc), as might be expected, there was an increase in errors where the product is labeled with incorrect instructions. This may be because staff had become complacent about the labeling process as a result of the robot implementation, even though the automated dispensing system had no effect on the labeling process, done through the pharmacy system.

These facts suggest that the difference in dispensing error rate reduction between these two centres is possibly due to a different baseline profile of dispensing errors in each department. However, in both cases, these figures would be confounded by the rate of dispensing errors for those items that were not dispensed by the robot, where the error rate would not be affected by the implementation of the system. Nevertheless, for both of these implementations, the error rate is greater than the absolute error rate cited by the Welsh researchers [17].

• Dispensing Process Efficiency

A number of efficiencies in the dispensing process have been observed in system evaluations. At the Wirral, an increase in the number of items dispensed per pharmacy technician per hour was observed, from 10 to 12 items per technician per hour prior to system implementation, to 15 + items per technician per hour after system implementation. The optimised dispensing process at the Wirral meant that the number of technician-hours in the dispensary had been reduced, with a corresponding increase in the number of technician-hours involved with near-patient services on the wards. This was equivalent to the redeployment of 3.5 wholetime equivalent (wte) pharmacy staff.

At Wolverhampton [8], dispensing process time allocation data were collected for two similar 2 week periods, one immediately before system implementation (August 2003) and one six months after implementation (May 2004). These data indicated that, not surprisingly, the time spent labeling and dispensing items was reduced, and the time spent restocking the machine was reduced, compared to stocking conventional shelves. However, the time spent on performing final checks was increased. Nevertheless, the net effect of these time reductions was that, after the implementation, the total number of items dispensed was increased by 19 %, and the total time spent by staff in the dispensary was reduced by 19 %. This latter figure was equivalent to the redeployment of 2.4 wholetime equivalent (wte) staff.

In surveys of pharmacy staff attitudes to the implementation of pharmacy robots in both the US [18] and the UK [9], it has been observed that, as might be expected, pharmacy support staff are more concerned than pharmacists about the impact of pharmacy automation on their job security. The possibility of redeployment may therefore be seen as a threat by pharmacy support staff. However, such redeployment enables pharmacy managers to utilise the best skill mix within the pharmacy team. Thus, the dispensary would have support staff operating the robot, with an accredited checking technician providing the final dispensing check, technicians would run the medicines management service on the wards, and pharmacists would work predominantly on clinical activities. As far as possible, all pharmacist clinical checks of prescriptions should take place on the wards (where it is easier to query issues with clinicians, patients, clinical notes and other patient management systems). This is the way in which re-engineering of pharmacy services throughout the hospital is made possible by the introduction of automation in the dispensary.

It might be expected that pharmacy robots would improve prescription through-put in the dispensary. The Wolverhampton team analysed dispensary throughput using data from their pharmacy tracking system before and after system implementation. They found that, while there was an increase in the number of items being dispensed in under 2 h, and a decrease in the number of items taking longer than 2 h to dispense, the overall impact on dispensary throughput was modest. In a similar way, the Wirrall implementers found that there was only a slight improvement in dispensary throughput, expressed as the cumulative percentage of prescriptions completed.

This modest change in throughput, despite implementation of a robot, may be due to three possible causes:

(a) There has been a general increase in pharmacy workload during the robot implementation period
(b) While the robot is processing prescriptions more efficiently, there has been an increase in pharmacy workload specifically due to the adoption of medicines management services, as these reduce bulk supplies, but increase the number of individually dispensed items.
(c) While the robot introduces efficiencies in prescription labeling, picking and assembly, there is still a requirement for a technician final check on the dispensed item. In a busy dispensary, this may become the rate-limiting step of the process, and may limit the potential of the robot to speed up the dispensary turn-around time.

It has also been noted that, following introduction of the robot at the Wirral, the time spent ordering medicines has decreased by on average 1 h each day.

It was suggested in the "Spoonful of Sugar" report [1] that use of automated dispensing systems as a tool for re-engineering pharmacy services would engender increased job satisfaction for pharmacy technicians, by releasing them to be involved in more clinically-focussed activities. However, research conducted on staff attitudes to pharmacy automation before and after a robot implementation [9] suggests that the implementation of automation does not have a significant effect on perceived job satisfaction.

• Use of Space in the Pharmacy

A major driver for introduction of automated dispensing systems in several centres has been the need to reduce shelf space in the pharmacy and to optimise the use of space. At both the Royal Free Hospital, London [10] and St Thomas' Hospital, London [6], installation of a robot led to more efficient use of space in the pharmacy department.

The effect of robot installation on space use in the pharmacy department was an important factor in the Wolverhampton system implementation [8]. In their analysis, the footprint (floor space) of the required pharmacy storage space after the installation of the Consis device was 10.2 m^2 (equivalent to 7 m^3 of space), compared to 14.3 m^2 (equivalent to 9 m^3 of space), prior to the installation. This space saving was significant in a dispensary with a total area of 77.2 m^2. At the Wirral, it was noted that robot installation led to the reduction of dispensary shelf space by 70 %.

It is clear that automated dispensing systems have a number of potential benefits, which have been quantified in detail in some centres. However, as with all automated systems, there are also risks associated with these systems. It is essential that potential implementers are aware of these risks, and that the systems are not promoted to staff as being "risk free".

The following issues and risks have been noted with automated dispensing systems:

1. In the early days of system use, many of the systems would dispense the required items, but would not apply the labels automatically. This meant that a human operator was still required for some of the dispensing process, and that labeling errors were not reduced by the use of the system. This effect is seen in the observed error rate for incorrect instructions on packs at Wolverhampton. This issue has been largely resolved due to the development of "in-line" labeling with pharmacy robots – i.e. where the label is applied in the robot as part of the automated supply process.
2. Downtime can occur due to broken bottles, lost bottle caps and split packs in the machine.
3. Not all medicines may be stored in pharmacy robots. The potential for service re-engineering and risk reduction is limited by the amount of pharmacy stock still requiring manual dispensing. Again this was a prominent issue when pharmacy robots were first introduced but has become less significant as pharmacy automation companies have developed CD and fridge storage facilities. However, systems still may not be able to handle large or bulky packs reliably.
4. Not all products have appropriate barcodes. At present, around 90–95 % of pharmaceutical products have barcodes – products such as clinical trial medicines, specials, parallel imports and some hospital packaged medicines may not be barcoded.

Evaluating the Benefits of Pharmacy Robots

As automated dispensing systems are, in effect, pharmacy departmental systems operating in a relatively discrete environment, their effects on operational risk are not as complex as with some other healthcare IT solutions, such as electronic prescribing systems. The various methodological issues and confounding factors in evaluating electronic prescribing and prescribing decision support systems are well documented [19], and have led to a call for standardisation of methodology used to evaluate such systems [20] (see Chap. 3).

There are currently few published papers providing a quantitative performance analysis of individual pharmacy automation implementations. It is to be hoped that more healthcare providers publish quantitative data on the performance of their pharmacy robots, in order to share experience with hospitals that are still considering the implementation of such technology, and also to enable pharmacy managers to formulate benchmark performance and risk management data for pharmacy robots.

This will provide a baseline analysis for robot performance while robots are still discrete, departmental systems. In the future, when pharmacy robots are interfaced with systems beyond the pharmacy (for example, electronic prescribing systems, oncology management systems, or wholesaler systems), other factors will confound the analysis of robot performance.

The Welsh Academic Pharmacy Practice Unit was commissioned to produce a toolkit for the evaluation of robot performance [21], and this has helpfully produced guidelines for research parameters and endpoints when performing a quantitative analysis of robot performance. They are shown in Table 4.2.

Analysis of the performance of individual automated dispensing implementations, and publication of the results, will provide information to help other hospitals refine the use of their robots. The availability of quantitative data will also ensure that the stand-alone benefits of pharmacy robots are fully understood before interfaces with other systems become widespread.

The extent to which estimated benefits will be realised will depend on the way pharmacy automation is implemented in each specific hospital, and hospital pharmacy managers should consider their service objectives before embarking on an automation project. Nevertheless, it may be argued that, in general terms, the pharmacy service improvements relating to the use of automation envisaged in the Spoonful of Sugar report are now being realised in hospitals that have pharmacy robot implementations. It is to be hoped that pharmacy robot suppliers will continue to develop their systems and provide enhancements to meet emerging functional requirements as hospitals begin to work with re-engineered or decentralised pharmacy services.

As with electronic prescribing, there is a relative dearth of quantitative data on the benefits of pharmacy automation. It is important that hospitals conduct work to quantify the benefits of pharmacy automation and publish their findings. This will (a) provide evidence which will be helpful for other hospitals at the stage of putting together a business case for automation, and (b) ensure that the benefits of pharmacy robots are fully understood before there is any move to integrate them with other electronic medicines management technologies.

Electronic Ward Cabinets

The natural extension of the use of robots to dispense medicines in a pharmacy is the use of electronic ward cabinets to automate the supply of medicines at ward level. These cabinets provide secure individual storage for medicines used on a ward, and are able to control and record access to medicines by ward staff [22].

Table 4.2 Guidelines for quantification of pharmacy robot benefits

Parameter	Evaluation recommendation	Other comments
Dispensing incidents	Data on dispensing incidents should be collected, as error rate will be low	
Distribution incidents	Distribution incidents should be monitored on two separate 1 week periods pre- and post-implementation	
Dispensary turn-around times	Turn-around time data should be collected for inpatient, outpatient and discharge prescription items	It is difficult to get accurate timings for all inpatient dispensed items
Out of hours dispensing	Use of the robot remote dispensing function by on-call pharmacists should be analysed	The out of hours cost analysis should take into account cost of travel to hospital and time off in lieu (TOIL)
Stock control	Staff resources (cost and time) spent on stock-taking activities should be analysed pre- and post-implementation	
Dispensing rate	Dispensing rate data should be collected on three consecutive days pre-implementation and on two intervals of three consecutive days post-implementation	
Distribution workload	Data on time spent on different distribution-related activities should be collected for a 1 week period pre-implementation and a 1 week period post-implementation	Workload survey results should be compared with issue statistics
Support staff attitudes	The attitudes of pharmacy support staff should be surveyed by questionnaire and/or other methods	The design of the survey and methodologies used should be customised to the needs of the department
Ward staff attitudes	The attitudes of ward staff should be surveyed by questionnaire 6 months pre-implementation and 6 months post-implementation	
Outpatient satisfaction	Outpatient satisfaction should be surveyed by anonymous question-naire for two periods of 2 weeks, pre-and post-implementation	

There is considerable experience of the use of these cabinets, which have sometimes been referred to as "magic cupboards", in US hospitals, but their use is very much in its infancy in the UK. However, their use has the potential to resolve a number of the problems associated with pharmacy stock control at ward level.

Traditionally, the process of pharmacy stock control in a hospital ward or department has involved a regular top-up by a pharmacy technician or assistant. Each ward would have an agreed stock list, with an agreed stock level of each item. On a regular basis (daily or twice weekly), the pharmacy technician would visit the ward, review stock usage and arrange for the stock on the ward to be topped up. The stock would be sent to the ward in a ward box, and it would be the responsibility of the nursing staff to unpack and put away the stock.

There are, however, many flaws in this system. Different nurses might put medicines away in different places, so the actual stock level for the ward might not be apparent to either the nurse administering medicines, or the pharmacy technician arranging supply. Medicines may not always be stored in the most appropriate places. Nurses may not be able to find the item they are looking for, and call the pharmacy department – sometimes out of hours – to rectify the situation. Orders are made for the "missing" items and the ward then has duplicate stock. In addition to this, if cupboards are untidy, there may be errors in the selection of the medicine (especially if there are similarities in name and pack design). These factors lead to an increased risk of patients receiving an incorrect medicine or missing a dose of a medicine altogether, accumulation of unnecessary stock on a ward and a lack of information about what stock is on a ward, therefore making it hard to conduct medicine use audits and to identify medicine theft.

Electronic ward cabinets have the potential to address a number of these issues.

1. They have individual drawers for each medicine and access to the device is via PIN, swipe card, fingerprint ID or a combination. They therefore facilitate secure storage of medicines.
2. Many cabinets have a significant capacity and can hold typically 150–200 product lines.
3. They facilitate correct product selection by clearly identifiable compartments, with visual identification of the medicine on the front of the drawer and possibly barcode verification of the medicine placed in the drawer. Draws may be modular and can be built to different designs to fit different products. Stock locations, therefore, are clearly defined.
4. They will draw patient demographic and allergy information from the hospital patient administration system (PAS), and can therefore provide decision support for allergies at the time of medicine use. Cabinets may also be used to enable barcode medicines administration (BCMA), using a barcode scanner at the point of issue.
5. Cabinets enable accurate stock control in a ward location. The cabinets are topped up by pharmacy assistant staff, in a similar way to a traditional ward top-up, but they provide accurate control of stock due to the individualized issue of items and the defined locations. They therefore have the potential to

prevent stock-outs and inappropriate ordering by ward staff. They will also enable pharmacy staff to do a full, periodic stock check, and this is advisable at an interval depending on the stock turnover on the ward.

6. Cabinets have functionality to monitor expiry dates, if barcode product information is scanned at the point of cabinet stock-up. This is a useful feature to prevent product waste.
7. Cabinets can provide audit trails and reports on the booking out of items (what and by whom), which can be useful in dealing with incidents and resolving disputes.
8. Cabinets can provide medicine use support, providing additional instructions and warnings concerning the medicine at the point of issue.
9. Many units are able to store controlled drugs and other drugs of abuse.
10. These units can also be used to enable and control dispensing of TTO/discharge pre-labeled packs of commonly used medications such as analgesia, laxatives and antibiotics, depending on the specialty of the ward. This is a common practice on surgical and day case wards in the UK.

Electronic ward cabinets may be configured in a number of different ways to support medicines management on a ward:

1. They can be used to issue the stock for a ward to a traditional drug trolley from which medicines would then be administered to patients.
2. They might be used to administer medicines directly to a patient.
3. They could be used to support patient self-administration, where the cabinet would be configured to have a PIN or access code for each individual patient.

The mode of use of the cabinet would depend on the type of ward and the types of patients on the ward. Surgical wards require a smaller number of commonly used medicines, and a cabinet is often straightforward to stock and run on this type of ward, while providing a significant benefit in error reduction in product selection. On the other hand, medical wards will have a wider variety of stock medicines, and this may be more challenging for the stocking and maintenance of the cabinet. Cabinets have obvious benefits in emergency departments, in terms of preventing product selection errors in urgent situations, but staff may have concerns about speed of access to medicines.

Benefits of Electronic Ward Cabinets

Electronic ward cabinets have been shown to provide the following benefits in published literature:

- Reduction in the number of missed doses [23]
- Reduction in delayed medicines and medication administration errors [24]
- Reduction in ward stockholding [25]
- Reduction in time taken to administer medicines [25] (especially for controlled drugs)

As mentioned previously, automated dispensing cabinets have been implemented widely in the US, where their use is facilitated by routine unit dose dispensing, and where there is a need to closely control stock issue on an individual patient basis, for insurance reimbursement purposes. Data from the 2007 ASHP Pharmacy Informatics Survey indicated that, while only 10.1 % of hospitals have dispensary robots, 82.8 % of hospitals had automated dispensing cabinets [26].

Ray et al. [27] have studied the use of a point of use unit dose dispensing system at the University of California San Diego Medical Centre. They found that the system reduced the waiting time until first dose, reduced medicine administration errors, reduced staff time and costs, and enabled better use of pharmacist's time. Chapuis et al. [2] studied the use of an automated dispensing system in a US adult intensive care facility, studying 1,476 medicines administrations in 115 patients. They found that the error rate (total opportunity for error) was reduced from 20.4 to 13.5 % and the system was acceptable to nursing staff.

In the UK, Omnicell electronic ward cabinets are in use at the Christie Hospital, Manchester, and also Kings College Hospital, London, but by far the most extensive installations are at Guys and St Thomas's NHS Trust (see Fig. 4.2), with 30 machines installed across the two sites (Guys Hospital and St Thomas's Hospital) for pharmacy use, and 100 machines for supplies. The majority of the machines were rolled out during 2009, but a machine has been operating in the Accident & Emergency (A&E) Unit at St Thomas's Hospital since 2007. The use of automated cabinets constituted a major change for the hospital and, during the installation and roll-out project, 300 pharmacy staff and over 6,000 medical and nursing staff were trained in the use of the cabinets.

In order to assess the benefits at Guys and St Thomas's Trust, a stock list review was conducted after the cabinets had been installed for 1 year, and the following benefits were identified (Mandeman D, personal communication 2012):

• One year after installation, amount of stock wastage had reduced by 22 %
• At the end of the stock list review, stock outages and ad hoc orders were reduced by 12 %
• Out of hours stock enquires to the pharmacy were reduced
• Time spent by ATOs topping up the wards was reduced by 20 h.

Overall, the number of stock orders being processed increased by 50 % following introduction of the cabinets, yet these orders were being processed with less wasted stock. This indicates that the cabinets facilitate considerable efficiency improvements at ward level.

Implementation Issues with Electronic Ward Cabinets

The installation of automated dispensing systems (cabinets) at ward level represents a major investment for a hospital and also a major change in the working process at ward level. There are therefore many issues that have to be considered when they are installed.

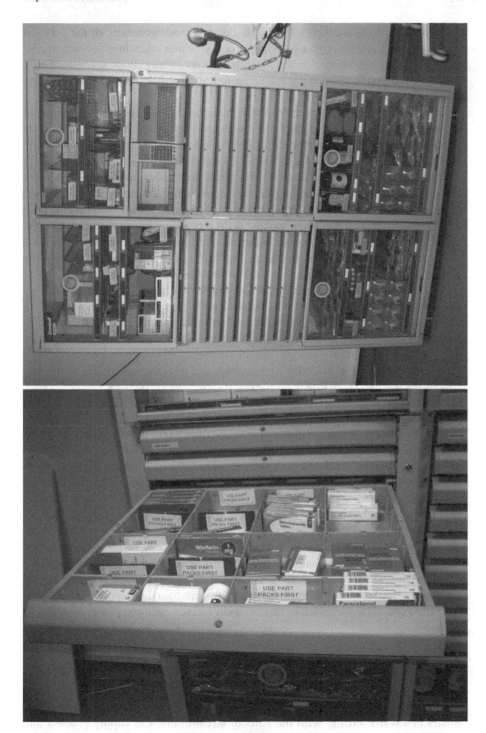

Fig. 4.2 Automated ward cabinets at St Thomas' Hospital, London, UK

There needs to be a process for installation and commissioning of the cabinets (cabinet installation and commissioning process) which takes into account appropriate operating conditions for the machine, power supply, floor space/footprint, ventilation, computer networking and communications (including wireless if necessary) and the layout of the working area.

There also needs to be an appropriate configuration for the ward cabinets, to determine how data exchange takes place with hand-held devices used by pharmacy technicians and the pharmacy system. Figure 4.3 shows the control architecture used for ward cabinets in the Guys and St Thomas's Trust.

Research should be done to establish how the devices will be monitored for benefits realisation, and to establish a baseline picture of stock control and movement on the ward. Managers should consider how the cabinets can be evaluated for possible benefits prior to procurement. This might include looking at the cabinets in operation at similar hospitals and evaluating their business cases, although there has been some research to suggest that some benefits of automated dispensing systems (for example, reduction of time taken to supply) may be evaluated using computer simulations of these devices [28].

As the installation of dispensing cabinets represents a major change in working practices for both pharmacy and nursing staff, early staff engagement, highlighting the benefits to those staff groups, is essential. A training strategy for nursing, pharmacy and medical staff is required, which ensures that locum, bank and temporary staff are trained in a timely and appropriate manner.

If the cabinets are used to enable barcode medicines administration (BCMA), the new working practice may be especially interruptive compared to the previous way of working. While there are benefits of barcode medicines administration (which are discussed in detail in Chap. 3), nursing staff will often find workarounds (BCMA work-arounds) to the barcode administration system, which will negate the benefits. These workarounds will include storage of medicines in places other than the cabinet, scanning a patient's barcode from their notes and not their wristband and many others. A study in a Dutch hospital setting [29] showed that barcode verification happened on only half of the medicines and that reasons for not scanning included problems with the scanning process (irregular shaped packs), lack of time, delays in computer responses and a lack of awareness about the importance of barcode scanning to patient safety. It is essential for project staff to be vigilant for potential workarounds that nursing staff may attempt, and provide training to address them. The problems of barcode workarounds could be resolved by training, engagement with staff to increase the culture of ownership of the system and dealing with technical issues such as improving wireless network coverage and considering a "hard stop" on the system to force staff to scan barcodes. The latter issue may be highly disruptive, but in certain settings might rapidly enable system compliance.

Remote Dispensing Systems

Automated dispensing cabinets are designed for operation by healthcare professionals in a ward setting, with the aims of streamlining the supply process and ward stock control. As such, these devices enable pharmacy services to be

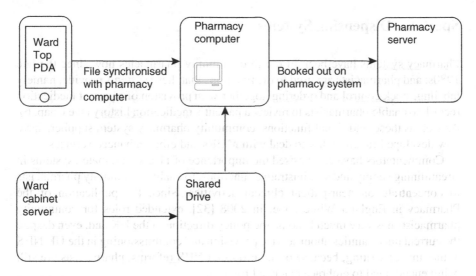

Fig. 4.3 Suggested ward cabinet control flowchart

decentralized from a central department and, as discussed, create the possibility of automated dispensing of standard discharge medication.

The next step is remote dispensing directly to patients, and automated kiosks have been developed to enable this. Automated kiosks enable medicines to be dispensed to patients against a prescription under the remote supervision of a pharmacist. They therefore can enable patient access to a pharmacy service at a hospital where there is no pharmacy department, or enable an out of hours pharmacy service. The use of automated kiosks has been explored for blood pressure monitoring and other telemedicine applications [30, 31].

The PharmaTrust MedCentre has been installed in hospital locations in Canada and the US and, while some British hospitals have considered the use of a kiosk, the law in Britain concerning pharmacist supervision of the supply of medicines currently precludes their use.

The patient inserts their prescription into the machine, or alternatively, the kiosk accepts an electronic prescription from a hospital electronic prescribing system. The patient pays for the prescription with cash or card, and the medicine is then prepared by the device. Patients then receive counseling from a pharmacist via a live video conference link.

The kiosk therefore provides the patient safety benefits of an automated cabinet (increased accuracy of product selection etc) and automated stock control, together with a pharmacy service, with advice and information available from a pharmacist.

Patient experiences of using kiosks have been positive, although conducting a remote consultation may require the pharmacist to develop new communication skills.

Specialist Dispensing Systems

Pharmacy systems have been in use in community pharmacies now since the late 1980s, and pharmacists are used to the functions that these systems provide, namely labeling, stock control and ordering, together with provision of a patient medication record, to enable pharmacists to review a patient's medication history (see Chap. 6). As well as these traditional functions, community pharmacy system suppliers have now developed functionality to deal with MURs and other enhanced services.

Commentators have emphasised the importance of IT and automated systems in streamlining supply and administrative functions, to enable community pharmacists to concentrate on near-patient clinical activities. Since the publication of the Pharmacy in England White Paper in 2008 [32], extended roles for community pharmacists has very much become the policy direction in the UK and, even despite the current uncertainties about service provision and commissioning in the UK NHS at the time of writing, because of the proposed NHS reforms, pharmacists are still being encouraged to embrace extended roles.

While automated dispensing using pharmacy robots is now common in hospitals, experience with automated dispensing in the community is less widespread. While automated dispensing would be beneficial in many larger community pharmacies, in order to deal with a high dispensing volume, the use of pharmacy robots has generally only been embraced by larger multiple pharmacy operators, and a number of independent community pharmacy innovators.

However, in addition to pharmacy systems and pharmacy robots, there are IT systems with the potential to support specific aspects of the community pharmacy service. An example of this is the use of IT systems to support methadone dispensing. A number of systems, such as Methameasure and Methasoft, have been developed to automate the dispensing of methadone to substance misuse clients in community pharmacies. Methadone dispensing and supervised consumption comprises an important element of a community pharmacist's work. In a national survey conducted to assess the impact of national guidelines on opiate substitution prescribing [33], it was found that, between 1995 and 2005, the number of prescriptions for opiate substitutes doubled, with methadone still making up the bulk of the prescriptions (>80 %). During the survey period, the average daily dose of methadone increased (from 47.3 to 56.3 mg), and the frequency of dispensing increased (from 38 to 60 % of prescriptions as daily instalments). During this period, supervised consumption has also been adopted (36 % of prescriptions in 2005). These factors have caused the volume of liquid methadone dispensing by community pharmacists to increase in the last few years and, despite the availability of other opioid substitutes such a buprenorphine, it is likely that the dispensing of methadone will continue to increase. Some community pharmacies dispense methadone for up to 300 clients per day [34].

Furthermore, as well as the volume of dispensing, there are a number of issues that make the supply of methadone a critical process, and which increase the risks associated with the methadone dispensing process in a busy pharmacy. Firstly, liquid methadone for clients with varying dose requirements must be dispensed extemporaneously, which is a time-consuming process. Secondly, in the UK, methadone preparations are Schedule 2 Controlled Drugs and their supply must be in accordance with the controlled drugs regulations (correctly generated prescriptions, maintenance of controlled drugs records, running balances and accurate dispensing).

Thirdly, the interpersonal factors with methadone supply are less straightforward that with other aspects of pharmacy practice. Because of their addiction, clients receiving methadone may dispute the quantity supplied and may use subterfuge and deception to obtain additional supplies. In addition, they may attempt shoplifting, which might place pharmacy staff under increased pressure to deal with them quickly so that they can leave the premises.

Consequently, the supply of methadone in community pharmacies is a prime area where robust procedures are needed to ensure that the supply process is efficient, legal and safe. It is recognised from studies of electronic prescribing and other medicines management IT systems that these applications can reduce clinical and professional risk, streamline working processes and enable better ways of working. Consequently, the process of methadone dispensing and supervised administration is therefore eminently suitable for the use of automation, where an automated system deals with the repetitive dispensing and record keeping process, allowing the pharmacist to deal with more intuitive aspects of the service – namely dealing with prescription anomalies and the client-facing supervision process.

A number of systems have been developed to automate the methadone supply process in busy community pharmacies where there are many methadone service users, and they consist of a computer-controlled measuring and dispensing unit. The software runs on a laptop computer and is attached to a cabinet containing two peristaltic pumps, one for standard methadone and one for sugar-free methadone. These pump the methadone from a bulk container to a dispensing nozzle, when the user selects a patient's methadone dose for dispensing. The pumps are highly accurate with a variance of less than 0.1 %, and the system maintains a running balance of methadone levels, from which printed CD register pages are generated at the end of the day.

Figure 4.4 shows the Methameasure system in operation at a UK community pharmacy.

Automated methadone dispensing systems offer the following benefits:

- automation of the dispensing process, thus saving time and reducing the potential for dispensing errors (especially in busy premises)
- no need to use bottles, when methadone is dispensed direct from the machine, thus reducing the cost of consumables.
- verification of client by photo record and/or fingerprint identification reduces the risk of dispensing incidents (either errors on the part of the pharmacy or attempts at deception on the part of the client)
- automatic production of controlled drug record documentation for the day, thus saving time for the pharmacist, and reducing the risk of discrepancies in the CD register.

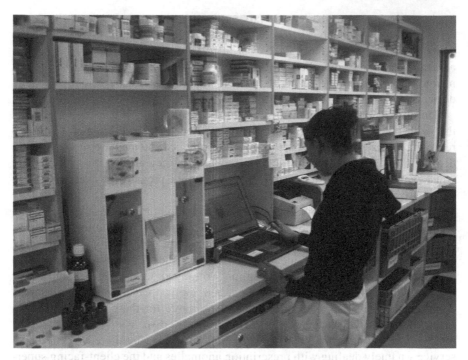

Fig. 4.4 Methameasure system at Cox and Robinson Pharmacy, Horsefair, Banbury, UK

A study has been conducted on the operation of the Methameasure system in ten pharmacies [35], but this study focussed primarily on financial savings in terms of staff costs and consumables, following introduction of the system, in order to help pharmacies formulate a business case for introducing the system. The study found that the average net saving afforded by installing the Methameasure system was £2,296.84. However, two pharmacies were excluded from the analysis, because the authors claimed that their data might skew the results, so the data were from just eight pharmacies.

With automated methadone dispensing systems, as with other medicines management IT applications, there is a need for large-scale quantitative data on broader system benefits, in particular the reduction of dispensing errors and the types of dispensing error reduced. Such data would contribute to a full understanding of the risk issues involved in the methadone supply process and would drive the adoption of these technologies as standard in high risk situations such as methadone dispensing. It is to be hoped that academic practice research pharmacists with an interest in this field might consider undertaking such work.

As with all IT systems used in healthcare, pharmacies installing automated methadone dispensing systems should check that the system meets all their likely requirements. For example, users may wish to check how flexible the system is with complex dispensing – for example, splitting daily doses, asymmetric dosing or changing installments during the prescription durations. Some of these use cases represent necessary control exerted by the system on the process but, in some cases, it may be possible to facilitate complex dispensing using configuration options in the system. Users should also check whether the methadone storage facility within the device complies with the legal requirements for storage of controlled drugs, and whether the system can be securely set up in patient consultation areas. Many systems now have secure storage on their devices, which conforms to legal requirements for the storage of controlled substances.

Conclusions

The use of automation has considerable potential to reduce risks of dispensing and supply errors and thereby improve patient safety. Automation can also improve the efficiency of the medicine supply and administration process, and improve the quality of services. Following the publication of the Audit Commission Spoonful of Sugar Report, pharmacy robots have been widely adopted in UK hospitals. However, there is still more scope for these units to be installed in the community pharmacy sector. Also, there is still little research information quantifying the benefits of pharmacy robots and, at a time when patient safety and service efficiency are of increasing importance to health providers, more studies would be beneficial.

Electronic medicine cabinets have the potential to reduce risks associated with medicine selection and administration on the ward, to improve stock control and management (with associated cost reductions) and to facilitate good medicines management. However, while use of these systems is widespread in other health economies, their use is still at an earlier stage in the UK, and there is little data on quantitative benefits, as yet.

Automated methadone dispensing systems are likely to have a beneficial impact on the efficiency, accuracy and safety of methadone dispensing in community pharmacy. The benefits of the system for the community pharmacist have been described, and there is an algorithm to assess the financial viability of the system in any given pharmacy. However, at present, there are no quantitative data available on the effect these systems have on the incidence of dispensing errors. These data would be beneficial for identifying risk factors in methadone supply, making standard operating procedures more robust and maximising patient safety.

References

1. Audit Commission. A spoonful of sugar – medicines management in NHS Hospitals. London: Audit Commission; 2001.
2. Chapuis C, Roustit M, et al. Automated drug dispensing system reduces medication errors in an intensive care setting. Crit Care Med. 2010;38:2275–81.

3. Swanson D. Automated dispensing – an overview of the types of system available. Hosp Pharm. 2004;11:66–8, 77.
4. Black A, Brice S, et al. Validation of cold storage shelves in an automated dispensing system. Hosp Pharm. 2006;13:372–4.
5. Brice S, Hardy L, et al. Evaluation of automatic loading devices with a ROWA speedcase system. Hosp Pharm. 2006;13:375–8.
6. Gross Z. Robotic dispensing device installed at St Thomas's Hospital. Pharm J. 2000;265:653–5.
7. Slee A, Farrar K, et al. Implementing an automated dispensing system. Pharm J. 2002;268:437–8.
8. Fitzpatrick R, Cooke P, et al. Evaluation of an automated dispensing system in a hospital pharmacy dispensary. Pharm J. 2005;274:763–5.
9. Coleman B. Hospital pharmacy staff attitudes towards automated dispensing before and after implementation. Hosp Pharm. 2004;11:248–51.
10. Anon. Royal free robot launch. Pharm J. 2003;270:359.
11. Anon. Robot will enable remote dispensing. Pharm J. 2003;271:438.
12. Taheri L. How clinical pharmacy services can be improved by pharmacy automation. Pharm J. 2012;288:335–6.
13. Clark C. Pharm J. Pharmacy Automation 2003;271:590–1.
14. Smith B. Using the Lean approach to transform pharmacy services in an acute trust. Pharm J. 2009;282:457–62.
15. Colquhoun A. Could automation improve efficiency and help pharmacies with cost saving? Pharm J. 2010;285:587–91.
16. Whittlesea C, Phillips C, et al. Automated dispensing – how to evaluate its impact. Hosp Pharm. 2004;11:283–5.
17. Whittlesea C. What did the research reveal about the effects of introducing automation? Hosp Pharm. 2004;11:453.
18. Crawford SY, Grussing P, et al. Am J Health Syst Pharm. 1998;55:1907–14.
19. Trent Rosenbloom S. Approaches to evaluating electronic prescribing. J Am Med Inform Assoc. 2006;13:399–401.
20. Reckmann MH, Westbrook JI, Koh Y, Lo C, Day RO. Does computerised provider order entry reduce prescribing errors for hospital inpatients? A systematic review. J Am Med Inform Assoc. 2009;16:613–23.
21. Whittlesea C, Phillips C. Automated dispensing – how to evaluate its impact. Hosp Pharm. 2004;11:283–5.
22. Green C, Hughes D, et al. Ward automation: an opportunity to improve the management of medicines. Pharm J. 2009;283:395–8.
23. Schwarz HO, Brodoury BA. Implementation and evaluation of an automated dispensing device. Am J Health Syst Pharm. 1995;52:823–8.
24. Borel JM, Rascati KL. Effect of an automated nursing unit based drug dispensing device on medication errors. Am J Health Syst Pharm. 1995;52:1875–9.
25. So J. Presented at guild of healthcare pharmacists Purchasing and Distribution Interest Group (PDIG), Ward Based Robotics, Birmingham, June 2011.
26. Pedersen CA, Gumpper KF. ASHP national survey on informatics: assessment of the adoption and use of pharmacy informatics in U.S. Hospitals – 2007. Am J Health Syst Pharm. 2008;65(23):2244–64.
27. Ray MD, Aldrich LT, et al. Experience with an automated point-of-use unit-dose drug distribution system. Hosp Pharm. 1995;30(1):18ff.
28. Tan WS, Chua SL. Impact of pharmacy automation on patient waiting time: an application of computer simulation. Ann Acad Med Singapore. 2009;38(6):501–7.
29. Van Onzenoort HA, Van den Plas A, et al. Factors influencing bar-code verification by nurses during medication administration in a Dutch Hospital. Am J Health Syst Pharm. 2008;65:644–8.
30. Houle SK, Chuck AW. Blood pressure kiosks for medication therapy management programmes: business opportunities for pharmacists. J Am Pharm Assoc. 2012;52(2):188–94.

31. Resnick HE, Ilagan PR, et al. TeahM – technologies for enhancing access to health management: a pilot study of community based telehealth. Telemed J E Health. 2012;18:166–74.
32. Department of Health (UK). Pharmacy in England. London, 2008.
33. Strang J, Manning V, et al. Does prescribing for opiate addiction change after national guidelines? Methadone and buprenorphine prescribing to opiate addicts by general practitioners and hospital doctors in England, 1995–2005. Addiction. 2007;102:761–70.
34. Scottish Chemist review. Methameasure of success. 2007:34–35. http://www.methameasure.co.uk/files/SCR.pdf. Accessed on Apr 2012.
35. Hand et al. Data on file. Methameasure Ltd. 2006.

Chapter 5
Electronic Medicines Management in Primary Care

For people in many countries, their predominant experience of healthcare will be of primary care, whether that is the general medical practitioner's consulting room in UK or European medical centres, the family physician's office in the United States, or through community pharmacies or nurse-led clinics in any of these settings. Throughout the Western world, many healthcare needs are met without the need for hospital referral, and the allocation of resources reflects that. In the UK NHS, prescribing in primary care accounts for around 80 % of the total medicines budget [1].

Given the sheer financial and human resources allocated to the primary care networks in many health economies, it is essential that systems used for enabling medicines management and pharmacy practice in the community ensure high quality of care, efficient use of resources and appropriate use of the skills of all professionals involved in the medicines user process. In particular, the relationship of the community pharmacist with other members of the primary care team is vital, and systems used for medicines management in primary care must support and enable this relationship, so that the pharmacist's unique knowledge and expertise is brought to bear to ensure high quality pharmaceutical care, and the minimization of adverse events.

This chapter will examine the functions of general practice (medical office) computer systems, in general but with a specific focus on the prescribing process, and also the process of electronic transfer of prescriptions (eTP) in the community, which is being adopted in the US, UK and other countries, and how the eTP process could support pharmaceutical care.

The Development of Systems for Medicines Management in Primary Care

In most developed countries, there is quite rightly a separation in primary care between the prescribing of medicines, which is done primarily by doctors, but increasingly by other health professionals [2], and the dispensing of medicines, which is done primarily by pharmacists, but sometimes by other agencies, such as appliance contractors. Increasingly, however, the distinction is blurred; in many countries, pharmacies are increasingly being located on the same site as medical practices, and in some cases medical practices are working with internet or mail-order pharmacies to supply medication.

Nevertheless, medical practices and community pharmacies have historically been distinct as institutions, and have been managed in different ways. This is why historically systems used to support medical and pharmacy practice in primary care have largely developed as separate entities.

In the UK, systems used in general medical practice (GP systems) have been in routine use since the 1970s. First and foremost, these systems enable doctors to maintain patient records to support good quality patient care and to ensure continuity of care, as well to provide a record of decision making for medicolegal purposes, as discussed in Chap. 2. GP systems also need to support the working practices of general medical practitioners, such as referrals to specialists, processing of test results and provision of contracted medical services (items of service) such as vaccinations and contraceptive services.

Clinical systems for medical practices in England are provided by the commercial sector, and are regulated by the GP Systems of Choice (GPSoC) initiative. The market leader in the UK, with 60 % of the market, is EMIS, but other suppliers include InPractice Systems (INPS)(Vision), iSOFT (Synergy and Premiere) and Microtest.

Traditionally primary and community care health professionals require patient record systems that have the following functionality [3]:

- To enable the clinical care of the patient by helping the health professional to structure the consultation and make appropriate decisions
- To provide a record of previous consultations
- To store and display test and investigation results
- To display referrals to and from other clinicians
- To enable sharing of patient information with other professionals who have access to the system.
- To enable the transfer of the record to another medical practice if the patient moves to another area

The GP system should also support the following activities:

- Epidemiology and public health monitoring
- Identifying target groups for screening and health promotion schemes
- Medical audit and activity monitoring (to support bids for service provision and to improve quality of care)
- Patient access and contribution to records
- Provision of medicolegal evidence in cases of medical negligence, or third party claims (e.g. occupational illness or pharmaceutical product complaints)
- To support social benefits claims
- To enable commissioning of community and secondary healthcare services
- To support health professional education and continuing professional development (CPD)
- To support clinical research and adverse event reporting

GP system records also need to be available to out-of-hours medical services, which provide a medical service to a locality during the evenings and at weekends, when GP surgeries are closed. There are two approaches to GP system access for out of hours services:

(a) a read-only system giving access to an external electronic health record system (for example, the Graphnet system)
(b) Read and write access to a single logical record – or separate records (e.g. TPP SystmOne and EmisWeb respectively)

There is an increasing trend towards centralized medical records derived from GP systems being accessed in other healthcare contexts by other healthcare professionals, as shared records. These are typically summary records containing minimum details (e.g. current medications, allergies, diagnosis and medical history), which are beneficial to support unscheduled care, typically in the out-of-hours (OOH) medical service, but also other services such as accident and emergency and community clinics.

These would include:

• Summary Care Record (SCR) in England
• Emergency Care Summary (ECS) in Scotland
• Individual Health Record (IHR) in Wales

Regional healthcare systems, such as those that have been established in Italy [4] and Sweden [5], enable a shared medical record to be used across primary care and unscheduled care settings. Some systems operated by US healthcare insurance providers – e.g. Veterans Administration (VA) and Kaiser Permanente – also provide a shared medical record for patient care in a number of primary care contexts (see Chap. 2).

There are potential benefits of shared records in terms of improving the quality of care in each care encounter, improved patient safety, improved access to care and better cost-effectiveness. However, there are risks associated with shared records, associated with record management and security, and responsibilities for maintaining the record. In the UK, the Royal College of General Practitioners (RCGP) has addressed some of these issues in its Shared Record Professional Guidance project [6]. This project elucidated a number of principles governing the use of a shared record (see Chap. 2), which covered:

• Obtaining consent to store and share data
• Clear assignment of clinical responsibility in care records
• Health professionals using records in a way that is consistent with their legal and professional obligations.
• Procedures for amending errors and offering differences of opinion in records
• Clear identification of the originator of any record entry
• Appointment of an information governance guardian for the organization.

In future, shared medical records may be used to support device integration and telecare (see Chap. 8).

Clinical Coding for GP Systems

While the importance of clinical coding and classification to support healthcare and medicines management activities has been discussed in Chap. 1, the development of coding systems to support general practice and primary care merits further discussion.

Pivotal to the development of GP systems has been the development of appropriate classification systems to ensure that information on diagnoses, treatments, interventions and other medical concepts can be transmitted between systems in a machine-readable way, which preserves the accuracy and semantic scope of the information. In the 1980s, computer systems were considerably less powerful than those used today, and the main reason for "coding" at that time was to reduce the memory required to store patient records, by replacing the full-text description of commonly recorded clinical concepts with short codes – typically four or five alphanumeric characters. Use of coding also meant that only a few characters needed to be typed for the complete text of matching clinical concept descriptions to appear on the screen for selection. This enabled the doctor to create a comprehensive record of a consultation on screen during the course of the consultation, without needing to be a proficient typist.

The most important clinical coding scheme developed for primary care in the UK was the Read Code system, developed by Dr James Read, a GP in Loughborough [3]. In 1987, the Joint Computing Group of the RCGP and GMSC adopted the Read Clinical Classification as the standard coding scheme for GP records in the UK.

Another important classification scheme used in medicine is the Systematised Nomenclature of Medicine (SNOMED) which was administered by the College of American Pathologists, and was derived from classifications of tumour and pathology nomenclature used by the College, which is in use in over 40 countries. SNOMED International (SNOMED III) incorporates almost all ICD 9 terms, so reports can be generated in ICD 9 format.

In 1999, the College of American Pathologists and the UK National Health Service announced their plan to converge SNOMED and Clinical Terms (Read Codes) v3 into a single terminology. The stated intention was to avoid duplication of effort and to create a universal, international terminology to support electronic patient records. The first version of the combined terminology – SNOMED Clinical Terms – was released in 2002, and was adopted as the standard terminology for UK NHS Connecting for Health healthcare applications [7]. Since 2007, SNOMED CT has been owned by the International Health Terminology Standards Development Organisation (IHTSDO).

It is likely that the NHS scheme of coding will migrate to SNOMED-CT over the next few years [3]. SNOMED-CT contains the same content (and more) but delivered in a technically different way. Implementation of SMOMED-CT will allow all parts of the health service to communicate and share data more reliably. For example, in a study comparing diabetes coding in primary care systems with the WHO classification for diabetes, SNOMED-CT was found to be more concise than 5-byte Read Codes [8]; with 5 byte Read Codes, 46.3 % of terms could not be clearly mapped to the WHO classification, but with SNOMED-CT, this was reduced to only 19.1 % of terms. Furthermore, it has been suggested that the use of SNOMED-CT in primary care systems would improve links to reference technologies for decision support [9]. However, Read codes are still the predominantly used coding scheme in GP systems at present, and SNOMED-CT would need to be used as the native coding dataset within systems (i.e. as the main internal coding system within the application) for it to be adopted more widely than at present.

Unlike disease classifications like ICD, Read Codes were never intended to be published in a hard copy format. For this reason, clinicians do not need to know what the codes are for different diagnoses, and some GP systems do not display the codes on the screen at the front end, although they are used for data processing by the system.

As mentioned earlier, a major problem with the use of coding and classification in GP systems and for transmission of information in primary care is that the code used has the appropriate semantic scope for the diagnosis or disease described. In coded records, there is often considerable variability, both in terms of what gets coded at all and in the particular codes chosen for the same clinical events at different times and by different users.

A significant cause of this problem is the way in which codes are presented to the user by the GP system, which may use alphabetical picking, default lists or "favourites" selection. Consequently, the design of the workflow of the GP system can lead to miscoding of clinical events and also perpetuation of miscoding by certain clinicians or within certain practices. There are also issues around code mapping when data are migrated to different systems.

All systems allow users to append text entries to Read-coded entries. Text appended in this way has the advantage that it is likely to retain its contextual relationship to the original Read coded entry even after record transfers to different systems. But this data may also become truncated or even lost by some systems following data migration or system update.

Text appended to Read coded entries should never change the meaning of the original coded concept. The UK Department of Health, BMA and RCGP guidance on GP systems [3] gives the following example:

G30.. Acute myocardial infarction excluded
would be strongly discouraged, while:
G30.. Acute myocardial infarction developed chest pain at work
would be acceptable.

Local codes are codes that are not part of the standard national code set (Read, SNOMED-CT) but which are generated at a more local level by a particular supplier, health community or practice. Local codes are usually generated to fill a perceived gap in the national dataset or to meet some specific local requirement. While some of these local codes, especially those that have been generated by system suppliers, may be essential to support normal system functions, they should not be used in preference to an established Read or SNOMED CT code.

Some GP system suppliers have embarked on programmes that automatically find their own local codes and replace them with Read or CT equivalent codes. These services are helpful for increasing the use of standard codes, and should be considered by practices. However, there may be instances where semantic assumptions are made by the code substitution process, and practices should be aware that these services will not necessarily reduce coding variability between clinicians and practices.

Some systems still allow users to create their own codes at practice level, but the use of unique practice-generated codes is not recommended. The semantic scope of the codes is often uncertain and there is variation in their applicability even in the same practice. Furthermore, these codes are rendered completely meaningless when transferred away from the practice.

Data Quality in GP Systems

Poor quality of healthcare data is an ongoing issue in the UK and indeed in other health economies [10], and the need for an improvement of data quality is well-recognised. This is as much the case with medicines-related data as with other clinical data. Pous et al. [11] studied 8 GP systems in Italy and found that the quality of medicines information in the systems was poor, and suggested various strategies for improvement. In a study of 3 GP practices in the north-west of England, Rogers et al. [12] found that there was no valid indication recorded for 14.8 % of repeat prescriptions, and that 62 % of the alerts generated by a GP system were incorrect.

In the UK, the PRIMIS Plus Project was set up to improve data quality in primary care by cascading multi-disciplinary information handling, and change management skills into individual practices. Data quality in the PRIMIS Plus project has been pragmatically defined as having five key attributes (represented by the acronym CARAT):

- Completeness
- Accuracy
- Relevance
- Accessibility
- Timeliness

GP System Functionality

Each GP clinical system has its strengths and weaknesses and different systems are designed to support particular styles of record keeping. It is essential that all members of the practice team have an understanding of the GP system that is commensurate with his or her role and responsibilities. Practices should ensure they have clear

policies supported by system-specific training for those users whose roles or responsibilities involve entering information relating to;

* Identifying patients/registration
* Problem and Episode Recording
* Recording Allergies
* Prescribing, Medication Records and Prescribing Decision Support Systems
  (DSS)
* Items of Service
* Pathology Tests
* Document Management/File attachments
* GP to GP Transfer
* Data Migration

Identifying Patients and Registration

GP systems have functions for recording various demographic data, including
patient name, address, gender, date of birth and healthcare identifier. This may be
an NHS number in the UK, or a healthcare maintenance organization (HMO)
identifier in the US. With GP systems, and indeed with pharmacy systems, it is
important that systems provide functionality to ensure identification of the patient
beyond reasonable doubt at the point of consultation. While a unique identifier
number may be the obvious way of doing this, numerical identifiers may not always
be available in systems or from patients, and a number of data fields may need to be
displayed to identify the patient fully. Adequate patient identification not only
reduces clinical risk, but it also improves data quality, as it avoids the creation of
duplicate records.

Problem and Episode Recording

Most GP systems are based on a problem-orientated approach although the detailed
implementation varies between systems. In all systems, problem titles are Read
coded concepts that describe the problems that the clinician has identified. These
problems may be:

* Diagnoses
* Major symptoms where a diagnosis cannot be confirmed
* Life events (e.g. bereavement)
* Major procedures (e.g. surgery)

Problem lists may be built from consultation records are made, or as information
is summarised from paper records, letters or reports. The goal is to build complete

and accurate problem lists. A particular problem will occur in an <u>episode</u> and episode types are usually classified in systems by the Royal College of General
Practitioners' classification of <u>First, New and Ongoing (FNO)</u>:

- First – signifies the first time the patient has presented with this problem in their
  life. There should be only one F episode for each diagnosis.
- New – signifies a new episode relating to diagnoses with which the patient has
  previously suffered but since recovered.
- Ongoing/Other – this designation is used when a patient attends and a health issue
  is discussed which is not a first diagnosis or a new episode of a first diagnosis

Consider the following example to illustrate the three episode types. A patient
might have more that one myocardial infarction (MI). The first should have an episode type "F" while further new MI should have an episode type of "N". However,
any episodes relating to an MI that has already been recorded, but that are not relating to a new/subsequent MI should have an episode type of "O". Failure to do this
can result in a record showing a patient has had more MIs than they actually have.

Each entry in the patient's problem list should represent a single episode of a
problem with an accurate date of onset. The data structure of systems is that Read
code can be used for all consultations about the same problem without adding new
episodes to the problem list.

However, GP systems vary in the way that they manage episodes (<u>episode man-
agement</u>). Some systems have functions that allow the user to maintain the quality
of the problem lists, and preserve the clarity of the consultation narrative, where the
view of encounter records can be filtered by problem title. This may involve:

- Linking problem titles with different Read codes to merge them into one episode,
  in cases where the diagnosis/problem is evolving.
- Correcting diagnostic or coding errors by deleting problem Read codes and
  replacing the deleted problem titles with correct Read codes without changing
  the meaning of previously recorded consultation records.
- Grouping related problems to make long problem lists clearer and enable a
  sequential view of a consultation (angina, myocardial infarction and ischaemic
  heart disease; or appendectomy and appendicitis) with the underlying pathology
  being the "group header".

Problems usually also have attributes of 'Active' or 'Inactive', which indicates
whether a problem is current, resolved or in remission. This allows for a further
structural level of 'episodes of care'. For example, 'Back Pain' as a problem may be
active or inactive many times during a patient's life.

Recording of Allergies

It is essential that clinicians realise that, for <u>allergies</u> to be transferable (interoperable)
across different GP systems, they must be entered in a way that interacts with the

native prescribing decision support system. Conversely, information relating to degraded adverse drug reactions in an imported record must be recorded in such a way that it interacts with their clinical system prescribing decision support software.

Transfers of allergy information between different systems may lead to problems because allergies can be handled in different ways in different systems. Not all systems use Read codes to record allergy information; some use other code sets to drive their prescribing decision support software. The UK medical data transfer project, GP2GP, has developed import mechanisms designed to recognise system-specific allergy information and then present the information to the user for action, during the data transfer process. However, some system specific information may not be easily mapped and will present as a text to be recoded by the receiving user. This issue is well-recognised and much work has been done to identify routines for allergy mapping which will reduce the amount of residual un-coded allergy data which falls out when data are transferred or migrated from one system to another [13].

Prescribing, Medication Records and Prescribing Decision Support Systems (DSS)

The prescribing of medicines was one of the first functions of early GP systems to be widely accepted. The use of the GP system for prescribing has been referred to some commentators as "electronic prescribing" but this is not strictly true as, in many settings, the GP system does not route an electronic prescription to a pharmacy, but simply generates a paper prescription, which is taken away by the patient. In future, however, the electronic transfer of prescriptions (eTP) from the GP system to a pharmacy system will become more widespread, both in the US with the development of community e-prescribing [14], and in the UK, with the roll out of the Electronic Prescription Service Release 2 [15]. Nevertheless, the advantages of using a GP system for generating prescriptions are similar to those for the use of EP systems. These include:

- Improved legibility of prescriptions
- Standardisation of drug names, packs and formulations
- Decision support for adverse reactions, contra-indications, interactions and duplicate therapy at the point of prescribing
- Specific warnings on controlled drugs and on high risk medication such as methotrexate.
- Standard orders for commonly prescribed items
- Medicine cost information is available to GPs at the point of prescribing and prescribing activity/medicine cost reports may be produced retrospectively.
- There is the potential for prompting for generic substitution in the workflow, which may be used to reduce prescribing costs. This will be discussed later in the chapter.

However, there are risks associated with prescribing using the GP system, and some of these are similar to those seen with hospital electronic prescribing systems. These include:

• The incorrect picking list selection for drug, dose or frequency selection.
• The prescribing of a medicine against the wrong patient record.
• Important decision support warnings not being actioned by the clinician
• Erroneous generation of repeat prescriptions (due to incorrectly set configuration options in the system)
• Instances when the item to be prescribed is not supported by the drug database on the system, and a handwritten prescription is required

Clinician prescribers should be trained in the use of GP systems for prescribing, and should take due care when using the system for prescribing. However, some of these problems can relate to the design of the system too, and pharmacists should be aware of this.

In GP systems used in England, the Dictionary of Medicines and Devices (dm ± d) is used to code medicines. dm + d is a medicines and therapeutics coding system based on SNOMED CT, and it is therefore being introduced to standardize medicine descriptions and enable intraoperability. dm + d supports a number of the NHS Connecting for Health initiatives, including the Electronic Prescription Service (EPS) for eTP, and the Summary Care Record.

Users will automatically generate the GP system medication record as they use the system to produce prescriptions, and these records should accurately reflect prescriptions produced by the system and subsequent actions in relation to prescriptions issued. However, to ensure that the medication record is as complete and accurate as possible:

(a) prescriptions should not be amended by hand if incorrect, but cancelled and a new prescription generated,
(b) prescriptions returned or not used should be destroyed and recorded as cancelled on the system,
(c) information on medicines not prescribed by the practice should also be recorded. These might include medicines prescribed by other healthcare professionals, over the counter medicines by the patient from a pharmacy and herbal preparations bought and taken by the patient.

There are a number of areas of prescribing that may be overlooked by clinicians when recording prescribing histories in GP systems. These include:

• Psychiatric medicines being managed by mental health teams.
• Chemotherapy being prescribed by oncology services
• Immunosuppressant drugs being managed in secondary care following transplant surgery or for the treatment of autoimmune diseases
• Clinical trial medicines.
• Homecare medicines

The GP system would therefore need to have functionality to indicate to the prescriber which medicines will be prescribed and managed by the practice, and which medicines will continue to be managed by other specialists and providers. The functionality would need to ensure that:

- All medicines the patient is taking are logged for decision support purposes (e.g. drug interactions)
- For medicines being managed by the practice, prescriptions should be issuable from the transfer of care date.
- For medicines not managed by the practice, it should not be possible to generate routine prescriptions for them

As well as decision support at the point of prescribing, work has been done on a range of systems to support the process of diagnosis and care pathway management. Decision support modules in GP systems may be useful in the management of chronic heart failure [16], identification of people at increased risk of osteoporotic fracture [17], and dementia diagnosis and management [18].

Items of Service

GP systems will have functions to flag up medical services for which the patient may be eligible on a proactive basis. This process is likely to involve an alert to the clinician, either at the beginning of the consultation workflow, or where the patient's record is accessed for some other reason.

Items of service might include:

- Vaccinations
- Cervical Smear Tests
- Contraceptive consultations

If the clinician believes that the patient is eligible for the service, and the patient wishes to receive the service, the system will guide the clinician through the consultation workflow for the service, which acts as an aide memoire to the clinician. If the service involves the prescribing of medicines, the prescribing function will automatically generate the relevant prescription(s). The system will then prepare, issue and/or transmit the reimbursement claim associated with the service.

Pathology Tests

Standards for laboratory investigation reports (pathology test results) were developed in the mid 1990s in the UK through the Pathology Messaging Implementation Project (PMIP), and they are now in universal use by GP computer systems. These message standards enable GP systems to receive pathology test results from hospital pathology systems. The PMIP message standards were developed for haematology, biochemistry and microbiology reports, but as similar standards have not developed in other disciplines, these reports have been adapted for cytology and radiology reports.

More recently, in 2005, a new pathology message set was developed in the UK to enable pathology tests to be requested electronically, and for all disciplines to be reported electronically.

PMIP messages usually identify the investigations conducted by Read codes but also permit un-coded investigations. Systems have offered facilities to allow practices to apply their own codes to these tests, but as mentioned above, practice self-coding is not be recommended because of the changes of meaning that it could introduce, and the data mapping issues that may arise with data transfer to another system, either for GP transfer or data migration.

The growth of web-based technology has provided a platform for other local systems for pathology test reporting. Clark et al. [19] described the use of Fountain, a front end for GPs in Tayside, Scotland, to enable them to easily access laboratory results for their patients.

As a result of the historical independence of pathology laboratories, there are many labs, which are conducting the same investigations, but reporting them using different units of measurement. Examples include the measurement of Haemoglobin concentration expressed in grammes per decilitre and grammes per litre. This presents an issue with data reporting from pathology systems and, while work is in progress to address these inconsistencies, this may take many years. In the meantime, this issue introduces clinical risk which is heightened by the increased transfer of data between systems – for example, the use of electronic GP to GP record transfers and centrally-hosted GP systems.

Document Management

Despite the increasing use of IT in healthcare, paper documents are still often used in primary care. A medical practice may need to generate letters of referral, reports to specialists and other third parties, letters of request and many more. Similarly, a medical practice will receive much external correspondence in paper form.

All GP systems have functions to provide integrated document management – for example the generation of referral letters from consultation notes and the prescribing record. Many systems also have the ability to scan, format and file hard copy documentation relating to the patient, in the same way that document management systems can do in other professional areas (for example, law or accountancy). While document management might be considered a "back office" function, the correct use of these functions within the context of the practice is pivotal to the safe and efficient management of the practice.

Practices would need to consider:

- What their policy is concerning scanning and electronic use of documentation
- How the system enables attachment of the scanned material to the EHR
- Whether and how the scanned documentation can be linked to the correct patient (preferably by use of NHS Number)

- What their policies are regarding <u>metadata</u> of the imported information and how dates are set

Document import functions need to take into account two important issues concerning medicines:

- How changes of medicine treatment cited in imported documents might be flagged to the clinician to enable changes to be made to records of repeat prescribing.
- How <u>adverse drug reactions</u> and <u>allergies</u> reported in imported documents are verified and logged onto the system in such a way as they will be retrievable and trigger clinical <u>decision support</u> functions, and not be lost in the import process.

GP to GP Transfer

All GP systems are designed differently with different data structures and data views and there is no straightforward way for the data from one system to be migrated to another system with 100 % accuracy and structural integrity.

In the UK, the <u>GP2GP</u> initiative enables electronic record transfer between GP practices. GP2GP record transfer is carried out using a <u>HL7</u> electronic message standard, which provides a common architecture into which GP system suppliers may map their data structures. This provides standard formats for encounter names and types, code mapping, test results and other clinical concepts. This allows records to be transferred in a form which is 100 % human readable and preserves as much of the structure of the record as possible, although will require some of the entries to be rekeyed to ensure structural accuracy in electronic form.

There are four particular aspects of current GP records where the record transfer process needs to be supplemented by additional rules or processes, to generate records that are fully usable and safe in the receiving system, two of which relate to medication [3]:

- Qualifiers – for example, some system forms carry qualifiers which are extracted as text. On import to another system, the forms cannot be reproduced so that the qualifier information appears as text
- Dates – for example, some forms carry contextualised dates (e.g. disease register forms) which will be degraded to text on import to another system.
- <u>Medication</u> – some medications (e.g. mixtures) cannot be represented in dm+d Where sender and receiver systems are different the details will be degraded to text
- <u>Allergies</u> – where drug details cannot be represented in dm + d and the sender and receiver systems are different, the details will be degraded to text

The main system supplier for <u>out of hours (OOH)</u> medical services (Adastra) offers an electronic document transfer of details of an OOH encounter and there is widespread use of this. However, it is text-based and so practices will need to encode this information de novo as if it were a paper-based communication.

Data Migration

When a new GP system is installed, there is a need to transfer (migrate) the data from the old system (the source system) and the replacement system (the target system), using software typically provided by different suppliers. This uses similar data transfer processes to those used in transferring data from one active GP system to another. In the UK, individual suppliers' data migration processes are assessed against a set of requirements developed by the Data Migration Improvement Project (DMIP), which provides a standard for data migrations between GP systems.

The data migration process should progress through the following stages;

1. Preparation and planning
2. Extraction of data from source system
3. Transformation/translation of data from source system format to target system format
4. Import of transformed/translated data to target system
5. Handling of exceptions and review of data in target system
6. Iteration as necessary of steps 2–5 until a satisfactory result is obtained at step 5
7. 'Cut over' to target system
8. Back-loading to target system of any data collected during the period of time from the final source system data extraction to target system 'cut over'
9. Review of information in target system in 'live'
10. Final sign off

GP System Safety and Usability

As the previous sections have indicated, the design of GP system functionality will contribute to both the safety and the usability of the system. As has been shown with hospital electronic prescribing, a safe system is one that facilitates the data capture, coding, prescribing, claims and communications processes in a way that minimizes errors, improves efficiency and enables new ways of working. However, the system also needs to be usable by the clinician at the point of care, and facilitate the consultation rather than hinder the process. These two factors are interrelated and may sometimes conflict with each other.

In a survey of UK GPs, Morris et al. [20] found that patient safety features in GP systems were considered important by GP users, but many were unsure what safety features their system had, and many had received no formal training in them. A similar situation has been observed with pharmacists and decision support/alert features in hospital pharmacy systems (see Chap. 6). Standards are required to ensure that high quality usable clinical decision support features were implemented in UK GP systems. Standards for clinical decision support have already been developed in the US to support electronic prescribing/CPOE.

Avery et al. [21] conducted a study to seek opinion from an expert panel on the most important safety features within a GP system. The following factors were identified as important features:

- Avoidance of spurious decision support alerts
- Making it hard to override clinically important alerts
- Having audit trails of activity when important alerts are overridden
- Support for safe repeat prescribing
- Support for call and recall management
- The ability to run safety reports

Avery and colleagues also emphasized the importance of a good user-computer interface. Of all the systems described in this book, GP systems are probably the systems used most closely during interaction with patients and there has been much research on how GP systems may be used appropriately within a consultation to facilitate the patient care process [3], for example, how patients might view their record as part of a triadic consultation.

The use of a GP system can have a negative impact on the consultation process, however. Studies have shown that GP systems may lead to reduced eye contact of GPs with patients and a reduced communication of information by the GP to the patient [22]. Refsum et al. [23] piloted semi-automated user action recording (UAR) software to analyse useability of two GP systems. Interestingly, they found that the system with the shortest time for the prescribing workflow had a longer time for the coding process, and vice versa.

Electronic Transfer of Prescriptions (ETP)

The electronic communication of prescriptions from a prescriber and a dispenser in primary care will be referred to here as the electronic transfer of prescriptions (eTP), as opposed to the term *electronic prescribing* (EP), which is used to refer to the electronic communication of prescriptions in hospitals. While some US publications (e.g. Fincham [14]) use the term electronic prescribing, or e-prescribing, interchangeably for both primary care and secondary care computerized prescribing, the systems and processes are still quite distinct in most economies and require separate evaluation. The author's view, therefore, is that a distinction should be made between the secondary care and primary care processes.

The electronic transfer of prescriptions has been enabled by regional and national healthcare IT systems in different countries, which include US insurance-funded systems, such as the Regenstrief Rx Hub [24], and systems operating in Sweden [5] and Italy [25]. In the UK, the electronic transfer of prescriptions was first tested in three pilots in 2000, which showed clear benefits for eTP [26]. As part of the NHS Connecting for Health programme, which was launched in 2002, the Electronic Prescription Service (EPS) has been established to enable eTP in England. With the

EPS, prescriptions generated by GP systems are transferred to the national spine, and can then be drawn down by a patient's nominated pharmacy.

The English EPS has been developed as two releases [27]. Release 1 of EPS (EPS Release 1) introduced the technical infrastructure to enable prescribers and dispensers to operate EPS. With Release 1, the prescription was still printed (which in itself is the legal entity) and it had a barcode. The pharmacy would scan the barcode, which would enable the prescription information to be downloaded to the pharmacy system from the NHS spine. However, the completed items were still be checked against the paper prescription (the legal entity) and the paper prescription was still submitted for reimbursement manually. Release 1 therefore provided some benefit in preventing re-keying errors in the pharmacy, but also provided the means to test the EPS infrastructure and system usability. Release 2 (EPS Release 2) abolished the need for a paper prescription, and enabled an electronic prescription containing an advanced electronic signature to be sent from the prescriber's GP system to the NHS Spine, which could then be drawn down by the patient's nominated pharmacy. Release 2 also enabled electronic cancellation of prescriptions, and electronic repeat dispensing which increases safety and the whole process is smoother if electronic repeat dispensing is used by the practice. Release 2 also allows electronic submission of dispensing endorsements as part of the prescription reimbursement process.

Some scenarios are not supported by EPS:

- Scenarios where the prescriber does not have access to EPS (for example home visits and out of hours)
- Personal administration of medication
- Private (non NHS) prescriptions
- Bulk prescriptions for a school or institution
- Controlled drugs
- When the patient chooses not to have an electronic prescription
- When the prescription includes an item that does not have a dm+d code.

Benefits of eTP

Electronic transfer of prescriptions provides the following potential benefits:

- Transmission of a complete, legible and accurate prescription from a prescriber to a pharmacy, thereby reducing the potential for errors and omissions in the prescribing and dispensing processes. However, it should be remembered that the accuracy of the prescription transmission process is controlled by the workflow design at both the prescriber and pharmacy end of the eTP process. There have been some issues with the English EPS where the dosage instructions have not been correctly transmitted. This issue has been addressed by the development of system functionality to resolve this issue, and will ultimately be resolved by the development of a national dose syntax model (see Chap. 1)
- Transmission of electronic prescriptions in a secure manner [28]. However, while eTP systems might have appropriate security features in place, the security of the prescription information may be compromised by its display and storage at either end. Organizational information governance arrangements are in place to deal

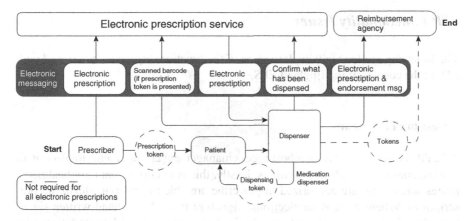

Fig. 5.1 Electronic transfer of prescriptions architecture

with this. Concern about patient information security, especially in the pharmacy setting, has been expressed in a UK survey of public, prescriber and pharmacist attitudes to eTP [29].

- Workflow efficiencies for the community pharmacy. Pharmacies can use an eTP system to streamline their throughput of repeat dispensing, to ensure that, for the majority of patients, medicines are ready to collect when the patient arrives at the pharmacy. The efficiency benefits that an eTP system can provide to the dispensing process can and should be used by community pharmacists to enable them to provide patient-focused services advice. The potential workflow benefits of eTP have been discussed in a recent review of the England EPS [30].
- Convenience to the patient in not having to submit a paper prescription to a pharmacy, and not having to wait for the dispensing process at the pharmacy. However, pharmacists will need to streamline their processes to ensure that waiting times are minimized.
- Provision of enhanced decision support functions to pharmacists. In theory, the availability of an electronic prescription should improve the triggering of decision support systems on the pharmacy system, and lead to improved patient safety due to an increased number of relevant alerts. However, there are no data at present to support this in the eTP/community setting.
- Provision of an effective communication channel between prescribers and pharmacists. eTP systems have the potential to create comprehensive communication channels between prescribers and pharmacists, to allow pharmacists to contribute to clinical care. However, the current England EPS system simply replicates the current prescription dispensing system, and does not allow for communication between professionals on any other clinical services.
- Enabling new working relationships. Fincham describes how eTP systems in the US can be used to change the dynamics of working between HMOs, medical providers and pharmacies [31]. However, as stated earlier, the current English EPS system is designed to replicate the current paper-based system, rather than to redesign it.

Figure 5.1 gives a flow diagram for the electronic transfer of prescriptions, based on the England EPS

eTP Functionality Issues

The following sections will explore some of the functionality issues associated with eTP in the context of the England EPS.

Access to eTP Systems

All eTP systems should have robust access management arrangements in place at all workstations in all healthcare settings. Firstly, this is to ensure that only healthcare professionals who are authorized to prescribe are able to generate electronic prescriptions. Where there is an electronic signature instead of a hand-written signature, there is a greater risk that unauthorized prescribing would go undetected by dispensers. Secondly, robust access management ensures that patients' prescription information is secure in any setting, and can only be accessed, viewed and acted upon by authorized staff.

Many systems use a password or password access control function. Biometric security (finger print or retinal scanning) has hitherto been too expensive to be scalable in a regional or national eTP system, but this situation may change. In the UK, the English EPS uses a Smartcard system to enable access to the service on the national spine. Smartcards are issued by what is known as a Registration Authority (usually the local Primary Care Trust), and new healthcare professionals who need access to NHS Connecting for Health systems need to contact the Registration Authority to apply for a Smart Card. EPS Release 2 uses the "single card" model of access – an individual Smartcard for each EPS Release 2 user. Users must not share Smartcards, or share access sessions. While the legal responsibility for prescribing and dispensing remains with the prescriber and pharmacist respectively, compliance with the NHS Care Records Guarantee requires there to be an audit trail of users of the national spine, to ensure the security and confidentiality of the spine data. In any case, healthcare staff should also ensure that there are appropriate security and access arrangements at workstations in their organization, to ensure the protection of confidential patient data. Staff passwords should be changed regularly and different grades of staff should have different access levels, allowing use of different functions.

System Requirements

With a regional or national system for eTP, the system will consist of three components: (a) a central data store or messaging service (e.g. national spine in England, ePharmacy message store in Scotland), (b) a communications infrastructure, and (c) local GP and pharmacy systems, which will provide the eTP functionality and connectivity with the national spine. With EPS, GP and pharmacy systems must comply with the NHS Connecting for Health Common Assurance Process, which provides data and security standards for the service.

Advanced Electronic Signatures

For an eTP system to be truly paperless, it must be able to transmit electronic prescriptions that are legally valid under the jurisdiction in which it operates. With hospital EP systems, inpatient medication orders constitute *orders to administer* medication. They are therefore not truly prescriptions, and therefore do not need to comply with the legal requirement that the prescription is signed by the prescriber.

However, in primary care, a prescription is required for prescribing medicines, and therefore the eTP system needs to be able to transmit a signed electronic prescription, which is legal in the jurisdiction of operation. The English EPS has met this requirement by using advanced electronic signatures for the electronic prescriptions issued in Release 2. Legislation and data standards for secure electronic signatures have been developed over the last 10 years or so to cover requirements of e-commerce or business to business trade. However, only recently has the POM order of the Medicines Act 1968 been amended to allow an advanced electronic signature on an electronically transmitted prescription.

The EPS uses a 256 bit advanced electronic signature. The electronic signature is unique to an individual user and is applied using the individual's NHS Smartcard and passcode. It is the application of the advanced electronic signature to the electronic prescription message that qualifies it as an electronic prescription.

Routing and Messaging of Prescription Related Information

The architecture of an eTP system should be designed to support the business processes it intends to automate. However, as already mentioned, the introduction of a eTP system could be used to re-engineer the medicine supply process, and introduce a new way of working.

The English EPS supports the following routing and messaging processes:

- The ability for a patient to nominate a dispenser (pharmacy or appliance contractor)
- The ability to send acute and routine (repeat) electronic prescriptions
- The ability of a prescriber to cancel an electronic prescription (but this may only be initiated by the prescriber)
- The electronic submission of reimbursement endorsement messages
- Record status of dispensing
- Submit dispense notification
- Electronic repeat dispensing.

Pharmacy Nomination

One of the key features of EPS Release 2 is that patients are able to nominate a dispensing location – a pharmacy, a dispensing medical practice or an appliance contractor. Patients may nominate up to three dispensing sites but, since they may not nominate more than one site of each type, in practice, they may nominate only one community pharmacy. Moreover, the nomination can be only be to a single pharmacy location, not to a chain of pharmacies.

Patients may make their nomination either via the prescriber, or via the pharmacy. Pharmacies will not be notified when they have been nominated or when a nomination setting has changed. The UK Royal Pharmaceutical Society has recommended that pharmacists should seek written permission from a patient concerning their pharmacy nomination, as is currently the case with repeat prescription collection services [32]. However, this may not be possible in some situations – for example, mail order pharmacies. Nomination of a pharmacy to dispense prescriptions requires consent on the part of the patient, in the same way that consent is required for medical treatment and healthcare service use, and is governed by the same professional standards.

A patient's prescriptions issued through EPS Release 2 will be sent to their nominated dispensing site. If the patient wants to nominate a different dispenser, they must tell the prescriber this at the time of the consultation. Patients can change their nomination at the prescriber's or dispenser's location at any time, including part way through a repeat dispensing cycle (although patients are advised to change their nomination at the beginning or end of a repeat cycle). Any prescriptions which have not been downloaded before the change of pharmacy will be accessed by the new nominated pharmacy. When a nomination has been changed, any prescriptions that have not yet been downloaded will be transferred to the new nominated dispenser.

With EPS, changes made to a patient's nomination settings are recorded by the system and Primary Care Trusts will have access to audit facilities to monitor this to ensure that the system is being used appropriately. Pharmacists will need to maintain an audit trail to show that they have captured, recorded and acted upon a patient's nomination request in a timely manner.

Prescription Tokens

With EPS Release 2, an electronic prescription is transferred from the prescriber to the dispenser, and a prescription token is given to the patient in paper form. The prescription token is not a valid prescription and must not be used for dispensing, but it acts as an aide memoire to the patient. A prescription token must be issued by a prescriber to a patient when using EPS Release 2 for repeat dispensing, but are optional for patients receiving one-off prescriptions.

Prescription Retrieval

With the English EPS, electronic prescriptions may be retrieved:

(A) By scanning the barcode on the prescription token presented by the patient (or entering the patient's name and then confirming their identity by checking their address and/or date of birth)

(B) By manually entering the prescription ID printed on the prescription token
(C) By routine automatic download from the national spine (for prescriptions from patients who have nominated that pharmacy)

The use of a routine download function within an eTP system, rather than downloading each patient's prescription as they walk into the pharmacy, enables the system to be used to manage the pharmacy workload proactively, and to ensure that patients' repeat prescription medicines are ready before the patient comes into the pharmacy.

An automatic download can be done once a day, either in the morning in readiness for the beginning of the working day, or before close of business in the evening. Alternatively, pharmacy users may make manual downloads during the day, before specific wholesaler order deadlines, or delivery schedules. These are ways in which an eTP system can be used to deliver pharmacy workflow efficiencies.

Dispensing Tokens

With the English EPS, patients may also be issued with a dispensing token when their prescription is dispensed. Dispensing tokens may be issued for the following reasons:

- When a prescription has been downloaded at a nominated pharmacy, but the pharmacy is not able to fulfil the prescription and the patient wishes to go to another pharmacy. The prescription is released back to the spine and the patient is issued with a dispensing token, so that the prescription can be accessed at another pharmacy.
- Where a patient has nominated a pharmacy and either pays prescription charges, or is exempt from paying prescription charges for a non-age related reason. The dispensing token is printed in order for the patient to sign and declare their exemption.

As with the Prescription Tokens, the Dispensing Token is not a legal prescription, and is not subject to the secure storage requirements for prescriptions. However as they contain personal information, they should be handled, stored and disposed in a confidential manner.

Supply of Medicines with eTP

With traditional paper prescriptions, patients would "identify" themselves by the presentation of the prescription. However, with eTP, patients who may not be known to the pharmacy staff may present in the pharmacy and ask for the supply of a prescription medicine with no form of verification. Pharmacists therefore should have a procedure for identifying patients who present in the pharmacy to collect electronic prescriptions. This may involve the patient confirming their address and/or date of birth, as they would do when collecting a prescription currently, or providing some form of identification, as when currently collecting controlled drugs.

Problems with eTP

There are various problem scenarios which may occur with an eTP system. These include the following:

- The patient arrives in a pharmacy looking for supply of their prescription, but their electronic prescription has been issued through a different system to that used by the pharmacy. This might happen with an EPS Release 1 prescription in an EPS Release 2 pharmacy in England, or where a Scotland ePharmacy prescription is presented to an English pharmacy in the north of England.
- A patient arrives in a pharmacy urgently needing to collect their prescription but the patient has previously nominated another pharmacy and their prescription has already been routinely downloaded there.
- The prescriber has cancelled the prescription (with EPS Release 2, if the patient presents with a prescription token, and it is scanned, EPS will give a rejection message, saying that the prescription has been cancelled).
- The prescriber has not yet sent the prescription to the eTP system.
- The prescription has been removed from the eTP central repository in accordance with prescription expiry or system housekeeping rules.
- Electronic prescription download speeds may be slow. This may be as a result of local system speed, communications/networking problems, or problems with the central spine. eTP services should have support systems in place to deal with software and communications problems. Ideally a single helpdesk should be in place to deal with all eTP related problems, wherever they are occurring in the system architecture.

It may be beneficial for eTP systems to have mechanisms to return downloaded prescriptions back to the national spine/central repository, so that the electronic prescription can be downloaded elsewhere at another time. If a medicine is required urgently, and an electronic prescription cannot be made available by the eTP system, pharmacists should consider making an emergency supply according to the legal provisions of their jurisdiction.

Supplementary Clinical Information

There is often a need to communicate other relevant information concerning a prescription from the prescriber, to the pharmacist and then to the patient. When prescribing and medicine supply processes change on introduction of an eTP system, there may be a need for prescribers and pharmacists to review how information is communicated to the patient.

For example, the right-hand side of an English prescription form is in some cases used for communication of supplementary information to the patient. This might include the patient's repeat prescription review date, date of last repeat authorisation, or instruction for the patient to arrange an appointment for monitoring tests. With EPS Release 2, the patient may not always receive a prescription token – with this written information – so pharmacists will need to provide information relevant to the clinical care of the patient, in cases where the information is required. One solution to this problem with EPS is that pharmacists could provide printed information by printing the dispensing token for the patient with the supplementary clinical information on the right hand side. The pharmacist could then reinforce the printed information with verbal communication, where it is deemed necessary. Customised print-outs of supplementary clinical information from pharmacy systems would also be helpful.

Professional Checking

Pharmacists have a professional requirement to ensure that "every prescription is clinically assessed to determine its suitability for the patient" [33]. eTP systems are only a method of delivering prescription messages from the prescriber to the dispenser and the same clinical problems can occur on electronic prescriptions, as with paper prescriptions.

Pharmacy systems may assist efficient dispensing and checking of a medicine by pre-populating an on-screen "prescriptions" with details from the prescription message, but this information is for inspection and verification by the pharmacist and the usual professional dispensing vigilance is still required.

Substitution

With eTP systems, prescriptions are issued electronically for products using standard product codes (dm±d in the UK NHS – see Chap. 1). A product will be described either at the product level (dm+d VMP level – e.g. Aspirin Tablets 75 mg) or at the pack level (dm+d AMP level – e.g. Angettes 75 mg Tablets (Bristol Myers Squibb)). If the product is described as a specific pack, the prescription will therefore include details of the specific formulation and manufacturer, and under UK law, the pharmacist is obliged to supply the product type specified. However, it may not always possible for a pharmacist to supply a specific generic product against a prescription, due to stock availability and other considerations. For this reason, generic product (VMP) prescribing should be encouraged when eTP systems are operational.

Labelling of Prescriptions

Once an electronic prescription has been downloaded, it will be displayed on screen, possibly as a facsimile of a standard prescription form. The user can then select each item for dispensing, amending the directions as appropriate, and produce appropriate labels for each item. Unless an appropriate terminology for dose syntax is in operation (this is still being developed in the UK) then any directions transmitted by the eTP system may not provide adequate instructions to the patient for using the product, and pharmacists may need to use their professional judgment to ensure that all products are appropriately labeled for patient use. Some of the issues around directions or other label attributes may be resolved by tools or configuration options available within the end user pharmacy system.

Accuracy Checking

Traditionally, the final accuracy check for a prescription has involved the pharmacist checking the final dispensed items and labels against the prescription.

However, with eTP systems, there will, in many cases, no longer be a paper prescription to perform the check against and, since the electronic prescription is the legal entity, the accuracy check must be performed from the unedited prescribing data from the system. This may be done from the on screen prescription facsimile, (although there are health and safety implications if a pharmacist is checking from a screen all day), or from a printed version of the electronic prescription information.

Owings and Out of Stock Items

eTP systems should have the means of flagging up out of stock items for owing supply. EPS Release 2 flags items as either "dispensed" or "not dispensed" or one of two intermediate statuses – "partial" and "owing". Partial cover instances where an item is partially dispensed, and owing is where one item on a prescription of two or more items is completely out of stock.

Dispense Notification

An eTP system will usually send a message to the national spine or central server to notify when a medicine has been dispensed at a pharmacy. Ideally, the dispense message should be sent when a patient collects their prescription, to close the dispensing loop.

Submission of Reimbursement Endorsement Messages

An eTP system will manage the claim process by submitting an electronic reimbursement endorsement message to the healthcare management organization (HMO) or payor. End user pharmacy systems will need to be configured so that the appropriate reimbursement codes are submitted with the message. With the establishment of eTP systems, there is a need to test the electronic reimbursement process to ensure that it is operating according to the drug tariff rules of the health service, insurer or payor before full roll-out of the system.

Cancellation of Electronic Prescriptions

An eTP system should have functionality to enable an electronic prescription to be cancelled – either by the originating prescriber, or by the pharmacist, in both cases giving a reason why the prescription has been cancelled or not dispensed. Systems should have some mechanism to prevent a pharmacist downloading an electronic prescription that has been cancelled by a prescriber. Good communications between prescribers and pharmacists will be necessary to ensure that confusion does not arise in handling cancelled prescriptions. Ideally, systems should enable two way electronic communications between pharmacists and prescribers for prescription-related information.

Electronic Repeat Dispensing

eTP systems can enable a repeat dispensing process, which is laborious using paper prescriptions and, for this reason, was not readily adopted with paper prescriptions in England. With EPS Release 2, the prescriber issues a repeatable prescription, which is transmitted to the national spine in the usual way, and the patient is issued with a Repeatable Prescription Authorising Token. The system manages the release of each repeat issue. The first issue is available to be downloaded from the spine as soon as it is sent to the spine. Each subsequent issue is available once the previous issue is complete. The system will automatically send the next repeat issue to the pharmacy 7 days before the expected issue date of the next issue. Alternatively, a pharmacy can pull down repeat issues in advance of them being sent automatically by the spine, when the instalment interval is flexible.

Also, with EPS Release 2, patients can change their nominated pharmacy midway through a repeatable prescription. When a patient changes their nomination, any outstanding repeat issues which have not already been downloaded will be transferred to the new dispensing site.

Pharmacy systems may be configured to support different scheduling methodologies for repeat dispensing.

Data Structure and Product Selection

Due to potential product data mapping issues between an end user system and an
eTP system, a situation may arise where an item cannot be prescribed via eTP
because it has not been mapped in the GP system to the appropriate code. In these
cases, a paper prescription would need to be issued. Pharmacists may also identify
incorrect data mapping, usually where the item selected on the pharmacy system
screen does not correspond with the information printed on the prescribing token. In
addition, some product names may not display correctly on labels, because of the
implementation of codes in pharmacy systems. There needs to be an appropriate
error reporting system for these mapping issues, mediated either by the eTP system
supplier or by healthcare provider organizations.

Business Continuity

As with all IT systems, there will inevitably be times when an eTP system is unavailable. The causes of system failure with an eTP system will fall into three broad
categories, corresponding to the components of the eTP system:

1. Failure of the local pharmacy system
2. Failure of communications – telecommunications and/or internet connections
3. Failure of the eTP system national spine or central server

   While system failure and outage can happen with any system, it is particularly
critical with a delocalized system such as an eTP system. There is therefore a need
for a robust support and call-logging system for dealing with eTP system outage.
eTP systems or individual pharmacy systems may have tools to enable workarounds
in the event of system failure – for example default printing of electronic prescriptions, to enable a traditional method of prescription processing.

Adoption of ETP

Unlike IT developments in secondary care, hampered by stakeholder buy-in, funding and health service politics, there is a clear commercial imperative for eTP and
clear benefits to pharmacy operators, given the need to streamline the community
pharmacy workflow and the reimbursement of prescriptions. Furthermore, there are
corporate bodies such as community pharmacy multiples, wholesalers and community pharmacy software suppliers who are able to invest money in eTP systems.

However, experience with the EPS in England is that implementation of eTP has been slow. The take-up of EPS Release 1 was not as widespread as hoped; only 31 % of pharmacy sites were "business live" in mid 2007 and a year later, when the UK government wanted pharmacy contractors to move on to Release 2, many had not even begun to use Release 1. There were a number of factors behind the delay in eTP adoption. Firstly, there was little engagement with community pharmacists in the early stages of the project. While the business processes of EPS replicated existing pharmacy processes, they did not specifically support improved processes or new pharmacy roles, which were envisaged by pharmacy policy at the time. Consequently, pharmacists were reluctant to engage with EPS as they felt that the system was being imposed on them by the Government, and were not convinced that the EPS has been designed to serve their best interests. Secondly, the medical profession was initially reluctant to embrace EPS, even though they had the software capability and have been given funding to do so. The reluctance of GPs to move forward with the EPS was undoubtedly because some doctors felt threatened by pharmacists taking on new roles and encroaching on their territory.

Thirdly, there were issues with the coordination of stakeholders in eTP. In some areas, pharmacies were "technically live" with eTP functions on their pharmacy software, but medical practices are not ready, or willing, to move ahead with EPS. In other areas, GPs had adopted EPS software and are issuing bar-coded prescriptions, but pharmacies were not engaged with the EPS. In a few areas, both surgeries and pharmacies had the technology to run the EPS, but the local PCT was not ready to implement EPS in their area.

Prescribing Management Software

The growth of the primary care trust (PCT) network as payors in the UK, the availability of networked GP systems, managed by the PCTs, and the development of new web-enabled database platforms have made regionalized management of prescribing data a possibility. In the US, large healthcare providers such as Veteran Affairs (VA) and Kaiser Permanente have in-house proprietary systems to collect data on prescribing activity and drug use. However, in non-insurance based health economies, collection of prescribing data from a range of individual providers can be problematic, without standard data sets.

In the UK, where GP systems are managed by PCTs, there are systems for extracting and aggregating prescribing data. Data to support the Quality and Outcomes Framework (QoF) is extracted from GP systems to the Quality Management and Analysis System (QMAS) by the NHS Information Centre. There are also prescribing management systems which are interruptive to the prescribing process, and provide decision support to clinicians on choice of medicine, in relation to the local formulary. In the UK, Scriptswitch is used by 138 PCTs to provide prescribing decision support to GPs. Where implemented, the system provides substitution recommendations, based on agreed local NHS guidance. The system also provides dose optimization information and patient safety actually warnings. Scriptswitch also has reporting tools to monitor the number of switches that actually take place.

Furthermore, the development of web-based database platforms has enabled the development of commissioning information systems to enable commissioners to monitor activity, performance and payment of provider organizations. These look at total tariff service provision, not just drug use, and so provide a picture of the total expenditure relating to a therapeutic intervention.

Sollis provides a solution, Clarity PBC, which covers:

- Budget management – actual against budgeted, forecast outrun, variance analysis, performance alerts, high cost patient alerts
- Activity analysis – elective activity, non-elective activity, A&E attendances, consultant to consultant referrals
- Invoice validation – to match recorded activity against invoice claim
- Benchmarking – comparison of individual practices against regional or national average(s).

Sandhill Systems has produced Dune, a "cloud" solution for commissioning information, which can display information through any browser enabled device, and so does not require a specific software installation.

Conclusion

GP computer systems have been in use for many years to help primary care clinicians manage their practices. Prescribing and the management of medication-related patient information are key functions of these systems, and pharmacists should be aware of how they operate. A number of countries are looking at the possibility of the electronic transfer of prescriptions (eTP) in primary care, which offers benefits of secure prescription transmission, improved patient safety due to reduction of transcription and dispensing errors, and workflow efficiencies for both prescribers and pharmacies. However, it is important that eTP systems are designed to enable community pharmacists to take their place as a valued member of the primary care team. With the advent of sophisticated web-based systems and cloud computing, there are now systems with the capability of managing medicines use and claims data across organizations, in order to support the medicines commissioning process.

References

1. Picton C, Morris S. What you need to know about prescribing, the "drugs bill" and medicines management. National Prescribing Centre; 2008. www.npc.nhs.uk/resources/nhs_guide_for_managers.pdf. Accessed on Sep 2012.
2. Anon. Non-medical prescribing. Drug Ther Bull. 2006;44:33–7.

3. For discussion, see Department of Health, Royal College of General Practitioners, British Medical Association. The good practice guidelines for GP electronic health records. 2011, v4, p. 174. http://www.connectingforhealth.nhs.uk/systemsandservices/infogov/links/gpelec2011. pdf.

4. For example, the Umbrian regional healthcare system in Italy (see Barbarito F. Regional service card health and social care information system. Presented at opportunities in e-Health, London, 30 Nov 2006).

5. Sjoborg B, Backstrom T, et al. Design and implementation of a point-of-care computerised system for drug therapy in Stockholm metropolitan health region – bridging the gap between knowledge and practice. Int J Med Inform. 2007;76:497–506.

6. RCGP Informatics Group. Shared record professional guidance report. 2009. http://www.rcgp. org.uk/pdf/Health_Informatics_SRPG_final_report.pdf. Accessed on Apr 2012.

7. NHS connecting for health electronic prescribing in hospitals: challenges and lessons learnt. 2009. p. 74. http://www.connectingforhealth.nhs.uk/systemsandservices/eprescribing.

8. Rollason W, Khunti K, et al. Variation in the recording of diabetes diagnostic data in primary care computer systems; implications for the quality of care. Inform Prim Care. 2009;17(2):113–9. Accessed on Apr 2012.

9. Farfan-Sedano FJ, Terron Cuadrado M, et al. Implementation of SNOMED-CT to the medicines database of a general hospital. Stud Health Technol Inform. 2009;148:123–30.

10. De Lusignan S, Van Weel C. The use of routinely collected computer data for research in primary care: opportunities and challenges. Fam Pract. 2006;23:253–63. for a full discussion of the use of primary care data.

11. Pous MF, Camporese M, et al. Quality assessment of information about medications in primary care electronic patient record (EPR) systems. Inform Prim Care. 2010;18:109–16.

12. Rogers JE, Wroe CJ, et al. Automated quality checks on repeat prescribing. Br J Gen Pract. 2003;53:838–44.

13. Zimmerman CR, Chaffee BW, et al. Maintaining the enterprise-wide continuity and intraoperability of patient allergy data. Am J Health Syst Pharm. 2009;66:671–9.

14. Fincham J. E-prescribing: the electronic transformation of medicine. Sudbury: Jones & Bartlett; 2009. p. 23–31.

15. Taheri L. Completing the prescription process in a virtual world – EPS release 2. Pharm J. 2009;283:175–6.

16. Toth-Pal E, Wardh I, et al. A guideline-based computerised decision support system (CDSS) to influence general practitioners' management of heart failure. Inform Prim Care. 2008; 16:29–39.

17. De Lusignan S, van Vlymen J, et al. Using computers to identify non-compliant people at increased risk of osteoporotic fractures in general practice: a cross sectional study. Osteoporos Int. 2006;17:1808–14.

18. Iliffe S, Austin T, et al. Design and implementation of a computer decision support system for the diagnosis and management of dementia syndromes in primary care. Methods Inf Med. 2002;41:98–104.

19. Clark DH, Carter W, et al. How often do GPs use rapid computer access to laboratory results? A description of 18 months' use by 72 practices in Tayside. Inform Prim Care. 2004;12(1): 35–9.

20. Morris CJ, Savelyich BS, et al. Patient safety features of clinical computer systems: questionnaire survey of GP views. Qual Saf Health Care. 2005;14:164–8.

21. Avery AJ, Savelyich BS, et al. Identifying and establsing consensus on the most important safety features of GP computer systems; an e-Delphi study. Inform Prim Care. 2005;13(1): 3–12.

22. Nordman J, Verhaak P, et al. Consulting room computers and their effect on general practitioner-patient communication. Fam Pract. 2010;27(6):644–51.

23. Refsum C, Kumarapeli P, et al. Measuring the impact of different brands of computer system on the clinical consultation: a pilot study. Inform Prim Care. 2008;16(2):119–27.

24. Simonaitis L, Belsito A, et al. Aggregation of pharmacy dispensing data into a unified patient medication history. AMIA Annu Symp Proc. 2008;6:1135.

25. Barbarito F. Regional service card health and social care information system. Presented at opportunities in e-Health, London, 30 Nov 2006.
26. Mundy D, Chadwick DW. Electronic transfer of prescriptions: towards realizing the dream. Int J Electron Healthc. 2004;1:112–25.
27. For full business processes of the England EPS, see NHS Connecting for Health. EPS Release 2. Business process guidance for initial implementers. 2009. http://www.connectingforhealth. nhs.uk/systemsandservices/eps/suppliers/guidance. Accessed on Apr 2012.
28. For discussion of eTP security issues, see Mundy DP, Chadwick DW. Security issues in the electronic transfer of prescriptions. Med Inform Internet Med. 2003;28:253–77.
29. Porteous T, Bond C, et al. Electronic transfer of prescription related information: comparing the views of patients, general practitioners and pharmacists. Br J Gen Pract. 2003;53(488):204–9.
30. Harvey J, Avery A, et al. A constructivist approach: using formative evaluation to inform the electronic prescription service in primary care, England. Stud Health Technol Inform. 2011;169: 374–8.
31. Fincham J. E-prescribing: the electronic transformation of medicine. Sudbury: Jones & Bartlett; 2009. p. 25–6.
32. Royal Pharmaceutical Society. Good dispensing guidelines. 2009. http://www.rpharms.com/ best-practice/good-dispensing.asp. Accessed on Apr 2012.
33. Royal Pharmaceutical Society. Professional standards and guidance for the sale and supply of medicines. http://www.rpharms.com/archive-documents/coepsgssmeds.pdf. Accessed on Apr 2012.

Chapter 6
Pharmacy Management Systems

Introduction

The development of <u>pharmacy systems</u> to support working processes in both hospital and community pharmacy has taken place over the last 40 years in the UK, US and other countries. For the purposes of this chapter, pharmacy systems are defined as computer systems designed specifically for pharmacy departmental use, with functionality for the management of pharmacy and dispensing processes, such as medicine <u>labelling</u>, <u>patient medication records</u>, <u>decision support</u> for <u>drug interactions</u> and other warnings, <u>stock control</u>, <u>ward inventory</u> management, <u>order processing</u> and functions to support <u>pharmacy manufacturing processes</u> in hospitals. Pharmacy systems are often referred to as <u>pharmacy information systems</u> in healthcare provider organisations in the United States, or as <u>patient medication record (PMR)</u> systems in UK community/retail pharmacy.

History and Development of Pharmacy Systems

One of the first pharmacy departmental systems was installed at the John C. Lincoln Hospital, Phoenix, Arizona in 1975, at a time when early computers were for office use only [1]. The implementers of this system found that the computer was a very good way of standardising manual procedures and improving efficiency.

Moore et al. [2] described the implementation and use of a early pharmacy computer system at the Ohio State University Hospital. The system offered:

- Patient profiles
- <u>Order entry</u>
- Unit dose cart fill lists (<u>ward stock lists</u>)
- <u>Pharmacokinetic calculations</u>

S. Goundrey-Smith, *Information Technology in Pharmacy*,   151
DOI 10.1007/978-1-4471-2780-2_6, © Springer-Verlag London 2013

With the system, 95 % of medication orders were conditionally entered by pharmacy technicians, prior to being verified by a pharmacist. The authors notes that the advantage of a pharmacy computer system was that it could receive information from other hospital computer systems, but the disadvantage was that it was reliant on other systems for patient demographic information, such as admission, transfer and discharge data.

Gouveia et al. [3] described the pharmacy system at the New England Medical Center, Boston, US, which was developed to improve the department's financial and operational performance. This system was a mainframe based system and offered functions such as patient profiles, order entry, unit dose logging and financial reporting and management. The authors indicated that the system had a positive impact on the department's performance.

The earliest pharmacy systems in the US were either based on an individual personal computer or, if the hospital was technologically advanced, on a terminal attached to a hospital mainframe. Until approximately 1975, pharmacy computer systems available supported single operations, but from 1975, systems became available which offered a range of integrated pharmacy functions within the one system [4]. The literature on pharmacy system development in the US in the 1970s and early 1980s has been reviewed by Knight and Conrad [5] and by Burleson [4], and the problems and issues associated with the implementation of the early systems have been described [6–8].

Similar pharmacy system implementations were made at British hospitals during the 1980s, although in the UK, hospital pharmacy systems were very much departmental systems and, with the exception of one or two centres such as Winchester [9], there were no whole hospital information systems installed in the UK at this time. The adoption of pharmacy systems by community (retail) pharmacies in the UK took place at around the same time. One of the key drivers for system adoption in the UK was the introduction of the legal requirement for printed medicine labels, which came in 1976 [10] in UK hospitals. While hospital pharmacy departments routinely typed labels at this time, this was a laborious process – especially if the medicine required detailed directions. Additional warnings (e.g. the British National Formulary cautions) were usually applied to bottles or packs as additional labels, but this made the pack look untidy. Consequently, the advent of computerised labelling, where all of the medicine details, directions and additional warnings could be printed on a single label, was a significant improvement in both hospital and community pharmacy practice.

Pharmacy System Requirements and Use

The pharmacy system enabled a patient medication record to be kept, which was important for community pharmacists as, prior to computerised systems, they had no other access to a patient medication record. The other chief purposes of a pharmacy system in both hospital and community were stock control, ordering and management. In hospital pharmacy systems, inventory management (ward stock list management) and drug use reporting are also needed, although there are various problems associated with these functions. The detailed functions of current pharmacy systems will be discussed at length in later sections of this chapter.

In the UK, while hospital pharmacy systems were developed as procured systems by companies such as JAC Computer Services Ltd or Ascribe Plc, many of the community pharmacy systems were developed by the pharmaceutical wholesalers, or subsidiary companies, with the express purpose of providing stock control functions, and were often provided free as a service to pharmacies by wholesalers. This has meant that community pharmacy system functionality has been primarily concerned with stock management and ordering [11], but this has also had implications for the development of these systems, and the customer dynamic, which will be explored later in the chapter. Because the community pharmacist does not have access to a detailed patient prescribing record and patient notes in the same way that the hospital pharmacist has, the role of the pharmacy system as a patient medication record (PMR) is a prominent one in community pharmacy.

There is little research concerning pharmacists' attitudes to pharmacy system functions. In a recent study in Finland [12], pharmacy owners were surveyed to find out what features of the pharmacy system were important to them. They regarded the following features as important:

- Tracking drug expiries
- Drug interaction screening
- Electronic pharmacy reference tools (medicines information), and
- Check lists for patient counselling.

The conclusion of this study was that features that would help pharmacists address health policy objectives and public health priorities were at least as important as those functions purely concerned with logistics and medicine supply. As will be seen, these features are commonly available on pharmacy systems marketed in different countries.

There is little published data on the usability of pharmacy systems, although this area has been newsworthy in the UK in recent years as pharmacy system suppliers have been redesigning their systems to make them compliant to the England electronic transfer of prescriptions (eTP) system, the Electronic Prescription Service (EPS). Since electronic systems for medicines management are sociotechnical systems [13] in that their total effect is dependent on the system, the user and the working environment that the system is operating in, the human-computer interaction is of importance in the usability of pharmacy systems, as with other systems. In a study of pharmacy system usability, Kirking et al. [14] have found that the use of a pharmacy computer system led to more drug-related problems being identified and followed up with prescribers, but did not appear to interfere with the pharmacist's patient counselling skills. The impact of pharmacy systems on identification of drug related problems is similar to that observed with the implementation of an electronic prescribing system at the UK hospital [15].

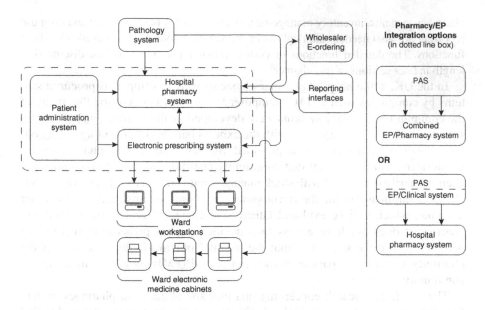

Fig. 6.1 Pharmacy system architecture in hospital pharmacy

Pharmacy System Architecture

Modern pharmacy systems will have a server/client architecture and, in hospitals will be integrated with other systems. A hospital pharmacy system will typically receive a feed of patient demographic data from the EHR or patient administration system (PAS) and may also have an interface with the pathology system to allow pharmacy users to view laboratory results, either when a prescription or chart is screened clinically or at the point of dispensing or labelling.

Increasingly, hospital pharmacy systems may be linked directly with electronic prescribing systems, and prescriptions for patients may be sent to the pharmacy electronically from wards and departments. Downstream from the dispensing process, the pharmacy system may have interfaces with a finance system, or with a pharmacy robot or other automated system (see Chap. 4), for full automation of the dispensing process. The system will also have some facility to export activity data to a reporting system to produce management reports of pharmacy workload and activity.

A hospital pharmacy system may therefore have the architecture (Fig. 6.1) shown above:

Community pharmacies also operate on a client/server basis often with a server for each pharmacy premises. However, the system will be fairly compact compared to a hospital pharmacy system, and many community pharmacies in the UK will have just one workstation. Larger pharmacies may have more than one workstation if they have a high dispensing workload, or if they manage a great deal of residential home dispensing, or supply of monitored dose systems for compliance (dosette boxes).

A recent issue in the UK has been concerning the method for processing prescriptions for the Electronic Prescription Service Release 2. The current procedure

Fig. 6.2 Pharmacy system
architecture for community
pharmacy

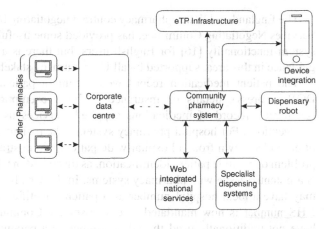

for paper prescriptions is that the paper prescription is used for the final check of the dispensed item. However, as discussed in Chapter 5, with EPS Release 2, the legal prescription entity will be the electronic prescription with an <u>advanced electronic signature</u>, so this should be used for the <u>final check</u>. This would entail the use of two workstations in every pharmacy – one to process the prescription and print the labels, and the other to conduct the final check. This would be required even in small pharmacies, and this has been the subject of some controversy among pharmacy contractors in the England, where EPS Release 2 is being rolled out.

The architecture for a community pharmacy system (Fig. 6.2) would therefore be as shown above, with links to eTP, other national services, pharmacy robots, specialist dispensing systems (eg methadone dispensing) and a corporate data centre, if a branch of a large pharmacy multiple:

Both the hospital and community pharmacy systems would have a secure internet connection to send automated <u>orders</u> to wholesalers. Electronic ordering and supply chain management will be discussed in greater detail in Chap. 7.

Community Pharmacy System Functions

Pharmacy systems provide a range of functions to support dispensing and pharmacy professional activity. These would include for a community pharmacy system:

- <u>Patient medication record</u>
- <u>Prescribing/Dispensing Decision Support</u>
- <u>Dispensing</u>
- <u>Labelling</u>
- <u>Stock control & ordering</u>
- <u>Product pricing</u>
- <u>Endorsement support</u>
- Support for other services.

The England and Wales pharmacy contract negotiating body, the Pharmaceutical Services Negotiating Committee, has provided some useful guidance on pharmacy system functionality [16] for English users, but there is a need for more detailed guidance in this area, supported by all UK pharmacy stakeholders.

The patient medication record would contain patient demographics (name, DOB, address), details of insurance or NHS exemption status (pre-payment certificate), record of medications supplied, services used and other pharmacy interventions. For hospital pharmacy systems, the patient demographic details are often pulled down from a hospital-wide patient administration system (PAS). The problem of positive patient identification, as discussed in Chap. 5 with GP systems, is a potential issue with pharmacy systems. In the UK, hospital pharmacy systems may have a local hospital number as a patient identifier, although the use of the NHS number is now mandated in UK hospitals. Community pharmacy systems have not traditionally used the NHS number as a patient identifier, but in some localities, pharmacies have keyed in NHS numbers to their systems to assist with service provision and monitoring.

Pharmacy systems have decision support functions at the point of dispensing, just as hospital electronic prescribing systems and GP systems have them at the point of prescribing. As with a GP system, pharmacy systems will alert the user to drug interactions, duplicate therapy, allergies and dose checking. However, they will also check the status of the prescriber and can provide a medication compliance check based upon the supply history. The system can also be used to record pharmacy interventions for the patient (queries to the prescriber etc.). Systems can be configured to print out decision support information – for example, drug interactions – onto labels to be given to the patient for information. However, these may not always be formatted in a patient-readable manner.

Pharmacy systems support the production of labels and other stationery for the dispensing process. As well as the labels for the medicines packs, systems can also print bag labels and labels for patient registration cards. Systems will also print medicines administration record (MAR) sheets and cassette labels for patients with compliance aids in residential homes and care facilities. Systems may also have the potential to print large print labels for the visually impaired. Systems usually allow pharmacies to design customised labels and print them using a thermal printer.

Systems will support all aspects of the dispensing process, including:

- Management of owings
- Instalment dispensing (e.g. methadone for substance misusers)
- Emergency supplies
- Private prescriptions
- Extemporaneous dispensing
- Repeat Dispensing
- Dispensing cycles for nursing homes

The system will also ensure that the correct reimbursement claim is made. In the UK, this relates to NHS prescription endorsement. Systems will apply the correct endorsement to a prescription based on current Drug Tariff recommendations, print the endorsement if a paper prescription is being processed, or make the appropriate electronic reimbursement message if eTP is being used.

Stock control functions are at the heart of community pharmacy systems; indeed, as previously mentioned, many of these systems were designed primarily for stock management. Systems will track and monitor stock levels and order processes can often be set for individual drugs. Systems will generate orders either manually or automatically, and send them via modem or paperless fax. Systems can be used to monitor best prices – for example, in the UK, current Category M prices for generics – and set up brand equalisation deals.

Systems should support pharmacy services other than dispensing, for example medicines use review (MUR), diagnostic screening and public health interventions [17]. For example, many UK pharmacy systems support the medicines use review (MUR) process to enable pharmacists to conduct MURs as an advanced service for the English pharmacy services contract. A pharmacy system will provide an on-screen MUR form, pre-populated with a patient's demographic details and medication history. The form would then guide the pharmacist through the review process and print the form and the GP notification report.

Hospital Pharmacy System Functions

The requirements for a hospital pharmacy system functions are similar, but with a number of more complex features. Hospital pharmacy system functionality would include the following:

- Patient medication record
- Product/bag labelling
- Controlled Drug Dispensing
- Stock control and location
- Stock ordering
- Stock costs
- Ward Stock Lists/Inventory Management
- Manufacturing Functions (Worksheets, Labels)
- Central Intravenous Additives (CIVAS)
- Total Parenteral Nutrition
- Chemotherapy

Many hospital pharmacy systems provide support for the latter three items listed above, but these modules may not always be used. It is common for CIVAS, TPN and chemotherapy to be outsourced to contract suppliers, manufacturers or specialist units, who will have their own IT systems and processes. Furthermore, if these services are provided in house, they may be supported by a specialist software package, either for historic or organisational reasons.

Another area that is often covered by private providers and therefore not covered in detail by pharmacy management systems is clinical homecare. Homecare is where low volume, high cost medication is produced in a customised manner, delivered direct to the patient, and administered in the home, usually by a health professional whose services are provided by the homecare company. While homecare is a growing market, NHS hospital pharmacists in the UK have had little involvement with homecare companies, and this has led to some controversy concerning the governance of homecare services. A review of homecare services has recently been done by the UK Department of Health, and recommendations have now been published [18]. While the benefits of homecare are acknowledged, the review has highlighted a number of shortcomings of the current homecare supply system. These include a lack of transparency in the commissioning processes, a need for more regional coordination and more governance from chief pharmacists of acute trusts. The review indicates that greater functionality to support homecare processes will be needed in both hospital electronic prescribing and hospital pharmacy systems, in order to strengthen governance and commissioning processes for homecare.

Many functions of a hospital pharmacy system are similar to a community pharmacy system, in terms of patient medication record keeping, dispensing support, medication warnings and stock control and ordering. However, there are three key areas where hospital pharmacy systems differ from community pharmacy systems:

1. Hospital pharmacy systems need functions for inventory management (ward stock lists) – to enable stock control not just in the dispensary(ies) but in the various wards and departments of the hospital. A hospital pharmacy system will therefore have various stock centres in its stock control database.
2. Hospital pharmacy systems are departmental systems of larger institutions, in the way that community pharmacy systems are not. There are more requirements, therefore, to interface hospital pharmacy systems with a range of other systems, such as electronic prescribing systems, pathology systems, pharmacy robots, electronic ward cabinets and other specialist systems.
3. While community pharmacy systems produce management reports for the pharmacy business, the hospital pharmacy system needs to produce a wider range of reports covering drug use audit and activity targets as well.

The next few sections of this chapter address these issues, and issue 2) is also discussed in Chap. 4 on pharmacy automation.

Stock Control Methodologies in Hospitals

There are a number of different approaches to stock control in hospitals. In the United States and mainland Europe, where healthcare payment is, in many cases, insurance-based, dispensing is based on unit dose activity, where each dose unit (tablet, capsule, suppository, vial, ampoule or aliquot of liquid) is packaged and dispensed individually to the patient, and charged to their prescribing record accordingly. For this reason, many of the devices for pharmacy automation (pharmacy robots, electronic ward cabinets etc.) introduced in the US or Europe have been designed to dispense individual dose units.

Traditionally, however, UK hospital dispensing has been on a pack basis, where a course of medication is supplied in an original pack, or a quantity of dose units is dispensed from a bulk pack (although there is now a move towards original pack use, because of the patient pack initiative, and to reduce the need for manual dispensing in pharmacies). As mentioned in Chap. 4, this "mixed economy" approach to dispensing has, in the past, acted as a barrier to UK market entry for some of the pharmacy automation manufacturers with established European markets, although systems for the UK market are now used almost universally.

However, the dispensing methodology in the UK means that the algorithms used for product costing and inventory control are more complicated for UK pharmacy systems that for those operating on a unit dose methodology. With unit dose dispensing, a single unit cost can be applied to each dose form, and prices of medication quantities issued may be easily calculated from this. With the UK hospital dispensing system as it has traditionally been, systems have to recognise pack sizes as well as dose units. If, for example, 15 amoxicillin 500 mg capsules are dispensed for a patient, then those capsules may be dispensed from a packs containing 15, 21, 50 or 100 capsules, and the user must select the pack from which the dispensed medication should be taken. As well as encouraging the usual problem of stock level errors, where an inexperienced dispenser takes the dispensed quantity from the wrong pack size, the presence of different pack sizes makes the costing functionality more complicated. Each dose unit will have a different cost depending on the cost of the pack from which it is taken, and often systems will assign a notional cost per dose unit to deal with this problem.

In the last 20 years, British hospitals have recognised that there are problems relating to inefficiency of supply and wastage of medicines in hospitals, due to the pack-based approach to dispensing. A number of approaches have been taken to address this.

Many patients come into the hospital with large quantities of their own medicines from home. Historically, when patients were admitted to hospitals, their medicines were reviewed and listed on the medicine chart or Kardex. Medicines would then be supplied to the patient from the ward stock or the pharmacy. However, because patient's own (PO) medicines cannot be used for another patient, large quantities of PO medicines were being disposed when a patient was admitted to hospital, even though they were often in perfectly good condition.

Therefore, in the 1980s many hospitals introduced use of PO medicines (patients' own drugs (PODs)) on wards, to ensure that these medicines were not wasted. A patient would bring in their medicines from home and, as part of the admission process, a pharmacy technician would check the PO medicines and, if the medicines were of appropriate quality, they would be used for the patient while on the ward. As well as reducing waste, this would eliminate the need for a supply of the medicine from the hospital pharmacy for the patient to use on the ward. With PO medicines – a medicine supplied by a community pharmacy, or a previous supply from the hospital pharmacy which has gone home with the patient – it is necessary to indicate both on the medication record and on the labelling that the medicine is a PO medicine. It may also be necessary to provide an additional label for a PO medicine, if the dose has changed on admission or if the original labelling was inadequate, while ensuring that the name and address of the original supplying pharmacy is still clearly shown. Hospital pharmacy systems should have features to support this process. PO medicines should be clearly marked in the medication record and allow appropriate labelling to be produced.

In recent years, problems have arisen around the process of discharging a patient from the hospital. There are financial pressures to reduce hospital stay times and increase bed turn-over. Patients need to be discharged from hospital with often a large number of medicines, and yet the information about medication changes from a traditional consultant's letter, sent by post, is not immediately available to the patient's family doctor in the community. From a hospital pharmacy perspective, the discharge process became inefficient because a patient was given a discharge prescription (or TTO (to take out) prescription) for their medicines to go home with, when often they had had a supply of their medicines on the ward only a few days earlier on admission.

For these reasons, a system of 28 day (one stop) dispensing was introduced in many British hospitals in the late 1990s. With this system, a patient's medicines would be checked on admission to hospital, and if there were any medicines that a patient was likely to be receiving on a long-term basis, a 28 day supply would be made for the medicine at, or shortly after, the patient's admission, fully labelled with directions for taking the medicine. This then provides the patient with a supply of a medicine which can be used in the hospital (and self-administered if appropriate for the patient) and then provide a supply of approximately 2–3 weeks for the patient on discharge. This process reduces the amount of dispensing required for a patient at the time of discharge, and helps to streamline the discharge process. However, the hospital pharmacy may need to relabel some 28 day dispensing items with new dosage directions, or supply additional items, at discharge. Hospital pharmacy systems should have features to support 28 day dispensing, ensuring that 28 day items are clearly indicated in the medication record, and that appropriate labels are produced. Systems should preferably have workflow features that facilitate relabeling of a 28 day item with new dosage instructions.

Another system that many hospitals have developed is an immediate discharge summary, to ensure that medication information gets from the hospital specialist to the primary care clinician in a timely way. This discharge summary may be in paper form, but is increasingly in electronic format, and is often also used as the discharge prescription. Pharmacy systems may need to provide an electronic interface to an electronic prescribing or clinical system generating discharge prescriptions or immediate discharge summaries.

Pharmacy System Interfaces

The market for pharmacy systems is now mature, and suppliers of both hospital and community pharmacy systems are looking to develop their systems in new directions. Hospital pharmacy system suppliers are looking to expand into provision of electronic prescribing functions, whereas community pharmacy systems suppliers are looking to develop features that support new clinically focused services. Both types of supplier are concerned with the development of appropriate interfaces with other systems. These issues are discussed later in this chapter. In addition, in the UK recently, the community pharmacy software suppliers have had to work closely with NHS Connecting for Health to enable to development of the Electronic Prescription Service (EPS) (see Chap. 5).

Hospital pharmacy systems have traditionally been departmental systems, but they are often interfaced with other systems within the hospital in a way that supports the pharmacy workflow. These will include:

- Hospital Patient Administration Systems (PAS) – to provide a feed of patient demographic information for the pharmacy system.
- Electronic Prescribing (EP) system – so that electronic prescriptions and orders generated in wards and departments can be processed.
- Pathology Systems – to enable pharmacy systems to receive and display laboratory test results pertaining to certain medicines (e.g. plasma levels with gentamicin or serum potassium with diuretics)
- Specialist Prescribing Systems – such as chemotherapy prescribing and manufacturing systems. This will allow the relevant pharmacy items – cytotoxic drugs, diluents, adjuvant agents and consumables – for a particular chemotherapy regimen to be booked out from pharmacy stock. This may also enable details of a chemotherapy regimen to be recorded against a patient's medication record
- Pharmacy robots – items are dispensed on the pharmacy system and then the issues are sent electronically to the robot as EAN/GTIN codes, so that the robot can pick the item. There may also be a facility for in-line labelling (i.e. the label is printed and applied to the item within the robot), or the label may be produced by the pharmacy system printer in the traditional way.
- Electronic ward cabinets – there may be a link to a server controlling automated cabinets in a ward or department, and also with a hand-held terminal to enable a pharmacy assistant to perform a stock/inventory check while on a ward. The mechanisms for this interface are discussed in more detail in Chap. 4.

The specific relationship between pharmacy systems and electronic prescribing systems is discussed in a later section of this chapter.

Reporting

The availability of activity reports is essential for business and service management and development. In the current financial climate, where health services are under pressure to become more cost-effective and productive, the role of reports as an indicator of current business activity and trends is becoming even more significant. Furthermore, with regular changes in the structure and initiatives of the health service, for example, the current proposed reforms of the NHS in England, there is a need for new and different report formats on a regular basis.

Pharmacy systems/PMR systems for community/retail pharmacy use will produce the following reports:

- FP34/Reimbursement Claim estimates – providing an estimate of the value of a pharmacy reimbursement claim
- Non-compliant Patient Reports – provides a list of potentially non-compliant patients and their medications, based on disparities between dose regimen and dates of supply
- Most Frequently Used Item Report – enables pharmacists to identify high use items (and costs) so they can look for and negotiate favourable deals with wholesalers and suppliers on these items.
- Residual Stock Reports – these reports would identify low, dead or excess stock, so that pharmacy managers can ensure that significant stock-outs do not occur and also that expensive stock does not accumulate on the shelves when it is not being used.
- Often Owed Products Report – in conjunction with the residual stock report, this can be used to identify products that are fast-moving, for which regular large orders should be made, to ensure patient/customer satisfaction.
- Prescription Throughput Report – this enables the pharmacy manager to keep track on the number of prescriptions being processed each day, to identify busy times of the day or week, and to plan staff rotas accordingly.
- Patient Histories – prescribing histories for individual patients may help to identify clinical problems with specific patients or to deal with complaints.

In secondary care and provider institutions, pharmacy managers often need reports from the pharmacy system to support prescribing and service provision targets, as well as to assess the productivity and commercial management of the pharmacy department. Some of these reports may be more recent requirements for the health service, but can be extracted from existing pharmacy systems [19].

Such reports may include:

- Directorate prescribing costs, for medical specialities
- Departmental activity reports
- Outpatient prescribing activity and cost reports
- Formulary compliance reports (prescribing of restricted drugs)
- Prescribing of drugs excluded from UK Payment by Results (PbR) (tariff costs)
- Compliance with HTA prescribing requirements (e.g. NICE in the UK)

These reports can be generated using reporting functions within pharmacy systems, or using reporting utilities and software [20].

Availability of Clinical and Medicines Information Through Pharmacy Systems

As discussed in Chap. 1, a range of medicines information reference sources are available for healthcare professionals. Historically, many of these were developed as paper-based reference books, but in recent years, they have been made available in electronic form, to support either stand-alone browser use, or use within a clinical system, either in an active or passive manner.

Various pharmacy systems (both community and hospital pharmacy systems) can be configured to make referential medicines information available within the pharmacy workflow. This might include:

- Summary of Product Characteristics/License Information
- Patient Information Leaflets
- Formulary Information (whether the drug is on formulary, or if it is subject to restricted use)
- Drug Interaction Information
- Use in pregnancy and lactation
- Off-label use

Another issue is the availability of dynamic clinical data, such as pathology test results, through pharmacy systems. Some literature [21] has highlighted the potential benefits of links between pharmacy systems and pathology/laboratory tests reporting systems.

These benefits would include:

- Increased evidence-based prescribing
- Improved dose adjustments
- Better monitoring of toxicity and
- Monitoring for drug interference with laboratory tests.

System Functions

Many pharmacy systems have been developed on a client–server architecture, but there is an increasing trend towards web-based systems, which provide greater scalability and ease of configuration. Such systems are beneficial in a large multiple pharmacy environment where there is a regular turn-over of premises on the estate. The web-based system can be mounted on a standard hardware platform in each premises. With pharmacy multiples, the configuration of the system across the business is significant. Some multiples have a separate pharmacy system in each premises, which may be interfaced with a central data centre, but in other multiples more of the system architecture is centralised at the head office

All pharmacy systems, regardless of their architecture, require a database structure that can manage the number of data items involved and the speed of processing – i.e. access to data for up to 60,000 products in a pharmacy that might be processing 1,000 items a day. Systems require regular software updates, and pharmacy managers should be aware of their system supplier's development road map, which should take into account forthcoming initiatives and trends in pharmacy practice.

Pharmacy systems should have drug data updates, to take into account the introduction of new medicines, the discontinuation of old medicines, changes to the warnings associated with medicines, and changes of tariff price. These updates should be delivered no less frequently than once a month [22] (because of price/tariff fluctuations) and may be delivered as a disk or, more commonly, as a modem update.

As with GP systems, there should be procedures in place to enable data transfer and migration from other pharmacy systems. This aspect is possibly more important with pharmacy systems than with GP systems because, in the UK at least, there are likely to be more frequent changes of ownership with pharmacy premises than with a GP surgery, and a new owner may require a change in system, especially if it is a multiple with another system established across the rest of its estate.

Community pharmacy systems require appropriate interfaces with external systems, such as eTP and other regional or national systems and initiatives. Issues specifically relating to the use of eTP services are described in Chap. 5. However, connectivity to external systems and services for pharmacy systems require compatible data structures, common messaging conventions and management of the data within a pharmacy system in a way that supports the system processes and data security of the regional or national service. With the EPS in England, pharmacy system interface is controlled by the common assurance process (CAP), where EPS technical specialists have been working with system suppliers to help suppliers to follow this process. There is also a need for community pharmacy systems to have links with other systems which support regional or national public health initiatives, although this is not always done in a consistent way. As discussed earlier, there is a need for hospital pharmacy systems to link with a range of other systems within the hospital to provide comprehensive functions to support both the operational and clinical aspects of hospital pharmacy.

As with any computer system for business use, a pharmacy system should have a comprehensive user help and support system, with on screen help, preferably at the point of use, and regular communications from the supplier about new system developments and how they can be implemented and configured.

Another basic requirement of systems is back-up, disaster recovery and business continuity. The system should have a regular on-site back up to disk, which is kept in a safe place, and also an off-site back up, in case of major disaster such as flooding or earthquake.

Benefits of Pharmacy Systems

There is little research information on pharmacy systems and the benefits and risks of using them (pharmacy system benefits). The pharmacy system market is mature and so, as discussed earlier in the chapter, much of the professional literature reporting pharmacy system installations as innovations dates back to the 1980s. A workflow study of an early pharmacy system implementation [23] indicated that the pharmacy system had a significant impact on departmental workflow, in terms of improving process efficiency. In addition, Croot et al. [24] indicated that pharmacy systems provided particular benefits to healthcare maintenance organisations (HMOs), where formulary control and information were key requirements. More recently, work by

Scullen et al. [25] indicated that an integrated medicines management system could enable significant cost savings and improvements in medicine use.

A recurring theme in the literature on pharmacy systems is the completeness of the pharmacy record in comparison to the prescriber's record. In a Danish study, Glintborg et al. [26] found that 6 % of prescription medicines prescribed for patients were not on the pharmacy record, 27 % of prescription medicines were not reported by patients when visiting hospital and 18 % of prescription medicines were not reported by patients on home visits. The authors indicated that it would be beneficial to review both pharmacy and prescribing records to prevent any medication errors arising from omission of medicines. Mabotowana et al. [27] looked at the use of pharmacy dispensing data along with GP prescribing data and concluded that a review of both datasets could improve the detection of patient adherence issues.

It is recognised that pharmacy systems contain considerable functionality for patient care provision that is often not used by pharmacy businesses and pharmacists may not input comprehensive patient data onto a pharmacy system, other than the record of prescriptions dispensed and patient allergies. Floor Schreudering et al. [28] conducted a study looking at the completeness of pharmacy patient records in Dutch community pharmacies and found that, in many cases, the pharmacy record was incomplete after the first patient visit. Only 67 % of all prescription drugs were recorded, no OTC medications, only 19.6 % of diseases and 3.7 % of allergies and drug intolerances were included on a patient's pharmacy system record after the first pharmacy visit. They concluded that pharmacists should be more proactive in collecting this data initially.

However, in contrast, it has also been recognised that the pharmacy record may contain information related to a patient's medicines that is not available elsewhere. Lau et al. looked at the completeness of hospital medication records [29] and found that 25 % of all prescription medicines taken by a patient were not recorded in the hospital medication record and that, for 61 % of patients, one or more drugs being taken were not documented in the hospital patient record. They compared these with community pharmacy records for the previous year and concluded that pharmacy records may help to fill the gaps left by GP records and patient recollection, and may also be used to identify "possibly used" drugs (those dispensed and might have been taken).

The relatively low levels of patient data in pharmacy systems may have implications for what decision support functions can be provided by a pharmacy system. Rahimtoola et al. [30] concluded that prescribers and pharmacists needed to share data as pharmacy systems had a limited decision support capacity on morbidity issues, due to a lack of disease data stored against patient records. In a Dutch study, Buura et al. [31] found that some diseases were recorded well on pharmacy systems, and some not so well, and that this has implications for the number of drug-disease alerts which can be triggered by the system.

In any case, recent work in the US has questioned the quality and usefulness of decision support features in pharmacy systems. In a study of pharmacists in Arizona, Saverno et al. [32] found that pharmacy systems were not reliable at identifying clinically important and relevant drug interactions – for example, serious drug interactions. Furthermore, another study in the same cohort of pharmacists suggested that pharmacists were not always aware of what decision support functions their pharmacy system had. Hines et al. [33] found that, while 60 % of pharmacists were aware of the drug interaction warnings that their system provided and 40 % were aware that not all drugs were included in decision support warnings, only 34 % were aware that their system provided pathology test result recommendations, and only 39 % were aware of paediatric dosage decision support on their system.

Because of the data fragmentation issues with the parallel use of prescribing and pharmacy records, there is a clear argument for prescribers and pharmacists, and indeed all health professionals, to have read and write access to a shared record.

The development of a common and complete medication record is possible with broad infrastructure systems, such as HMO systems like KP in the US. In particular, the Regenstrief medication hub [34], a HMO system in the US, combined an EHR with prescribing data with pharmacy claims (dispensing) data to produce a comprehensive medication record. In England, with the Summary Care Record and the Electronic Prescription Service, the English eTP (electronic transfer of prescriptions) service, it would be possible to produce a combined and complete medication record, and this is something that has been considered by NHS Connecting for Health.

Nevertheless, there are political factors involved with the use of shared records. In order to fulfil future professional roles in many economies, many pharmacists believe that they would need read and write access to shared records. As healthcare professionals, pharmacists are subject to codes of ethics and professional practice with requirements for safeguarding patient information. However, in the UK and elsewhere, access to patient records by pharmacists has been opposed by clinicians who may be concerned about the confidentiality of patient information in the retail pharmacy environment, but who may also be concerned that pharmacists are encroaching into their traditional roles. In addition, there have been concerns among patient and civil liberties groups about access to patient records by pharmacists. It is to be hoped that initiatives such as the UK shared record professional guidance project [35] will provide a procedural and ethical framework for shared medical record use by different healthcare professionals, and allow shared record systems to develop, where all professionals have appropriate read and write access to records. This will certainly help to resolve some of the problems associated with data fragmentation and omission of information in patient medication records.

Other Pharmacy Departmental IT Applications

Following the Noel Hall report in 1970, UK hospital pharmacy was restructured to enable the development of clinically-focused pharmacy activities, where the work of the pharmacist was concerned not just with dispensing medicines, but advising patients and other healthcare professionals on all aspects of medicine use. This would involve for example, therapeutic drug monitoring, producing guidelines for optimal patient treatment, management of specialist clinics and many other activities. This section describes some of these activities, and some of the IT solutions which have been developed to support them.

One area where IT systems have been developed to support clinical pharmacists is in the recording and reporting of data on pharmacy interventions (where clinical pharmacists query medicines use with prescribers and nurses), and the outcomes of these interventions. Data on pharmacy interventions are very important for hospital clinical pharmacy services, as they provide information on the medicines related problems being encountered in the hospital and also evidence of the activity levels and success of clinical pharmacists, both of which help to justify investment in clinical pharmacy. Systems which provide clinical pharmacy intervention logging will provide screens which will capture data on clinical interventions in a systematic way, tools for reviewing and grouping interventions, and automatic reporting of interventions. Intervention recording systems have been developed, for example, in Wales [36] and at the Antrim Hospitals in Northern Ireland (Beagon P. Antrim Hospital. Personal Communication 2011)] .

Nurgat et al. [37] describe the use of a web-based system for monitoring and tracking pharmacy interventions. With the use of the web-based system, it was identified that 29.06 % of pharmacy interventions led to cost savings (although this figure dropped to only 4.7 % when the system was being accessed on a multi-user PC). They found that the web-based system facilitated more complete data collection on pharmacy interventions.

Another area where various applications have been developed to support clinical pharmacy is pharmacokinetics – the study of drug absorption, distribution, metabolism and excretion (ADME). With the vast majority of medicines, the plasma level and metabolism of the drug does not have a significant influence on the efficacy or toxicity of the medicine. However, there are one or two drugs where there is a narrow therapeutic index and if the plasma level of the drug is too high the patient will experience toxic effects, or if the plasma level is too low, a therapeutic effect will not be achieved. With these medicines, the efficacy and safety of the treatment may be critically affected by poor dosing or drug interactions, and there is a need to monitor plasma levels in some or all circumstances (therapeutic drug monitoring). Such drugs include gentamicin, lithium, phenytoin and digoxin.

Since the metabolism of these drugs is described by mathematical algorithms, which have been elucidated in human pharmacokinetic studies of the drugs in question, software tools have been developed and validated to enable predictive monitoring of plasma drug levels by clinical pharmacists, so that drug therapy for a patient can be individualised and optimised.

As well as systems to support clinical pharmacy, specialist systems have been developed to support pharmacy manufacturing and quality control. Quality Management Systems such as Q-Pulse provide support for the quality management process, enabling production and retention of appropriate documentation, audit trails and reports for regulatory inspections and routine quality assurance. Companies such as Baxa provide systems for automated manufacture of total parenteral nutrition

(TPN) from individual ingredients according to bespoke formulae, and produce worksheets and audit trails.

Extension of EP Functions from Pharmacy Systems

As has been discussed in a previous chapter, electronic prescribing can provide considerable benefits in terms of (1) reducing the risk of medication errors (due to the electronic transmission of the prescription), (2) improving the medication prescribing and dispensing workflow in hospitals, and (3) supporting new ways of working in hospital pharmacy and medicines management. Nevertheless, adoption of functionally-rich hospital electronic prescribing systems is still at an early stage, even in the developed countries, due to the complexity of these systems.

An area that merits further discussion is the way in which a pharmacy system – handling pharmacy stock control – and an electronic prescribing system – providing electronic prescribing, decision support and electronic medicines administration on a ward – might be linked. There are two basic approaches. Firstly, the electronic prescribing functionality and pharmacy/stock control functionality may be two discrete modules of a larger hospital information system (HIS). This is the case with the Cerner Millennium system and the Meditech system, and is common in large US hospitals or health provider systems. This approach may lead to unhelpful dependencies on modules in other parts of the hospital, or problems if one set of functions is more advanced than another and there is a need for a third party supplier to meet the requirements instead of the relevant HIS module. Secondly, the electronic prescribing functionality may be an add-on module to the pharmacy system. With the demise of the England national IT programme, which had promised to provide a detailed national EP solution, the implementation of an EP from a pharmacy system provider may prove attractive to some UK hospitals.

The pioneering work conducted by a number of the US centres of excellence, such as the Brigham and Women's Hospital, Boston [38] has been enabled because these large teaching hospitals have considerable technical support in pharmacy informatics and coding. These resources are not universally available, and this is a barrier to EP implementation in some other regions of America [39], and also to smaller, local hospitals in all developed countries. A number of the earlier adopters of electronic prescribing in the UK, such as the Winchester & Eastleigh Trust [9], the Wirral Trust [40] and Burton on Trent [41] were able to install electronic prescribing as a module within a whole hospital information system. However, it is clear that, while the political will existed in these NHS trusts to enable these larges-cale IT implementations at the time, this approach cannot be easily replicated in other UK hospitals.

Nevertheless, the use of EP in hospitals may be enabled by the use of EP modules of established pharmacy systems. As they have the data structure, codes and domain knowledge, hospital pharmacy systems providers such as JAC and Ascribe have readily developed electronic prescribing modules for their systems. They have therefore been able to expand the market for their product by offering EP functionality to hospitals where their pharmacy system is in use, and also provide their customers with a potential "quick win" with adoption of EP functions. A number of UK hospitals have chosen to take this approach, for example, the Doncaster and Bassetlaw Hospitals [42] , the second generation Winchester Hospitals implementation [9] and the Birmingham Heartlands Trust [43] .

Fridge Temperature Monitoring Software

Some medicines need to be kept in a cool environment (2–8°C is the UK regulatory requirement) either while they are in the supply chain, or during their entire life. These typically include insulins, growth hormone products, desmopressin products and various others (although regulatory framework for storage requirements may vary from country to country). Pharmacy departments therefore need to maintain a cool environment for these products, and need to monitor the temperature of pharmacy fridges to ensure that products are being stored at the correct temperature and that their quality is not compromised.

Traditionally, pharmacy and ward fridges had analogue thermometers fitted, and pharmacy staff had to maintain a paper record of fridge temperatures. Twenty years' ago, this was a typical "start of day" task for junior pharmacy staff.

However, development of digital temperature probes has enabled the temperatures of pharmacy fridges to be recorded and logged electronically at pre-determined times, thus making the monitoring of pharmacy fridge temperatures a much less laborious process, and introducing the possibility of automated temperature alerts. Software has been developed to automatically monitor pharmacy fridge temperatures and make a detailed time-series record. The development of wireless, web-based systems means that fridge temperature monitoring can be done remotely, from a different location or out of hours, without the need for a dedicated PC to run the system.

Fridge temperature monitoring systems generally offer the following functionality:

- Routine temperature and humidity measurements at pre-defined time intervals
- Wireless sensors
- Alarms/alerts may be sent by email, text or bleep
- Alerts for out of range temperatures, loss of power or loss of data
- Flexible reporting options and formats for temperature logs generated.

Electronic recording of a temperature log for specific locations on a database system means that alarms and alerts can be configured for specific times, users and departments, and enables automatic calculation of industry parameters such as pasteurisation rates and dewpoint. A similar technological infrastructure – location probes/recording devices, database and web front-end – could also be used to monitor pH, pressure and other parameters.

Suppliers of fridge temperature monitoring systems include Icespy (Silvertree Engineering) and PharmaSlave (VVS).

Integrated Community Pharmacy Systems

As discussed, community pharmacy systems in the UK were developed largely by pharmaceutical wholesalers to enable stock control and ordering in the pharmacy. Originally, therefore, their functionality was primarily concerned with stock control, ordering and dispensing, and only recently have they been developed to support other pharmacy services.

Furthermore, while pharmacy systems for dispensary use were developed by pharmaceutical wholesalers, the electronic point of sale systems (EPOS)(cash registers) have been developed in the retail technology sector, are used in retail businesses of different types and are not specific to pharmacies. Consequently, in many community pharmacy businesses, there is no link between the pharmacy system in the dispensary and the EPOS/cash registers in the shop.

A number of system suppliers in the US and at least one supplier in the UK have developed a pharmacy system which is an integrated dispensing and EPOS system, and therefore can manage stock control and ordering across the whole pharmacy. With such a system, it is possible to assign details of medicines bought over the counter to patient's medication record, which could enable more complete medication records to be compiled. It is known that OTC medicine use is not recorded on pharmacy (and indeed GP) systems, and yet these medicines can interact with prescription medicines. Also with an integrated system, it is possible for an OTC purchase to trigger an alert within the dispensary system, and enable the pharmacist to intervene with certain sales on a consistent basis. However, with these integrated systems, the storage and use of EAN/GTIN item codes (EAN codes) for medicines is more critical to their operation as items will be scanned at the point of retail sale and be recognised by their EAN/GTIN code.

Systems to Support Clinical and Enhanced Services in Community Pharmacy

In the UK, Sonar Informatics has produced a series of web-based solutions to support the New Medicines Service (NMS), and other initiatives such as NHS (vascular) health checks and smoking cessation. A number of initiatives, managed by local Primary Care Trusts, are managed by Webstar, and have web-based forms and data entry screens. However, one of the barriers to full interface of these services with pharmacy systems is the lack of agreed datasets to support these services, and the fact that pharmacy system databases may not have the fields to support these datasets. This is an area of ongoing discussion and development.

Conclusion

Pharmacy systems were developed over 30 years ago, primarily to keep records of medicines supplied and to generate dispensing labels for medicines packs. However, these systems now provide a range of functions to support new roles for pharmacists and the latest developments in pharmacy practice. Hospital pharmacy systems may be interfaced with a range of other systems such as hospital EHRs, EP systems, pharmacy automation and other systems. Pharmacy systems are a valuable source of data for generation of reports to meet the changing management needs of pharmacy service providers. However, it is important that the views of practicing pharmacists are taken into account when pharmacy systems are designed and developed. Many other IT applications have been developed to support pharmacists with specific services and tasks.

References

1. Borggren L. Computers in pharmacy: improve efficiency and productivity. Comput Healthcare. 1984;5(7):39–40.
2. Moore TD, et al. The pharmacy computer system at the Ohio State University Hospital. Am J Hosp Pharm. 1984;41(11):2384–9.
3. Gouveia WA, et al. The pharmacy computer system at the New England Medical Center. Am J Hosp Pharm. 1984;41(9):1813–23.
4. Burleson K. Review of computer applications in institutional pharmacy – 1975–1981. Am J Hosp Pharm. 1982;39:53–70.
5. Knight JR, Conrad WF. Review of computer applications in hospital pharmacy practice. Am J Hosp Pharm. 1975;32(2):165–73.
6. Stroup J. Hospital pharmacy computer systems: request for proposal and the selection process. Can J Hosp Pharm. 1987;40(3):86–90.
7. Aldridge GK, MacIsaac D, et al. Managing the implementation of a pharmacy information system. Am J Hosp Pharm. 1993;50(6):1198–203.
8. Mildenberger J, Gouveia WA, et al. Managing the implementation of a pharmacy computer system. Am J Hosp Pharm. 1982;39(10):1692–701.
9. Goundrey-Smith SJ. Principles of electronic prescribing. London: Springer Science; 2008. p. 29.
10. Anderson S. Making medicines. London: Pharmaceutical Press; 2005. p. 143.
11. Taheri L. Completing the prescription process in a virtual world – EPS release 2. Pharm J. 2009;283:175–6.
12. Westerling AM, Haikala VE, et al. Logistics or patient care: which features do independent Finnish pharmacy owners prioritize in a strategic plan for future information technology systems? J Am Pharm Assoc. 2010;50:24–31.
13. Barber N. Electronic prescribing – safer, faster, better? J Health Serv Res Policy. 2010;15 Suppl 1:64–7.
14. Kirking DM, Ascione FJ, et al. Relationships between computer use and pharmacists' professional behavior. Drug Intell Clin Pharm. 1984;18:319–23.
15. Marriott J, Curtis C, et al. The influence of electronic prescribing on pharmacist clinical intervention reporting. Int J Pharm Pract. 2004;12(Suppl):R44.
16. See http://www.psnc.org.uk/pages/itsuppliers.html. Accessed on Feb 2012.
17. England and Wales contracted pharmacy services may be found at http://www.psnc.org.uk/pages/introduction.html. Accessed on Feb 2012.

18. Hackett M. Homecare medicines: towards a vision for the future. England Department of Health. 2010. p. 6–18. http://cmu.dh.gov.uk/homecare-medicines-review-group. Accessed on Feb 2012.
19. Davies A. Presented at the Guild of Healthcare Pharmacists/United Kingdom Clinical Pharmacy Association Information Technology Interest Group (ITIG) Seminar, Oct 2010, Birmingham. http://www.ghp.org.uk/ContentFiles/ghpitig10a.pps
20. Richman C. How to get useful information out of drug reports – and save time. Clin Pharm. 2011;3:186–8.
21. Schiff GD, Klass D, et al. Linking laboratory and pharmacy: opportunities for reducing errors and improving care. Arch Intern Med. 2003;163:893–900.
22. Royal Pharmaceutical Society. Guidance on pharmacy computer systems. London: Royal Pharmaceutical Society; 2003.
23. Sikora RG, Kotzan JA. Analysis of the change in work patterns following installation of an inpatient pharmacy computer system. Contemp Pharm Pract. 1981;4:160–6.
24. Crootof LM, Veal JH, et al. Pharmacy information system for a health maintenance organization. Am J Hosp Pharm. 1975;32:1058–62.
25. Scullin C, Hogg A, et al. Integrated medicines management – can routine implementation improve quality? J Eval Clin Pract. 2011. doi:10.1111/j.1365–2753.2011.01682.x.
26. Glintborg B, Poulsen HE, et al. The use of nationwide on-line prescription records improves the drug history in hospitalised patients. Br J Clin Pharmacol. 2008;65:265–9.
27. Mabotuwana T, Warren J, et al. What can primary care dispensing data tell us about individual adherence to long-term medication? Comparison to pharmacy dispensing data. Pharmacoepidemiol Drug Saf. 2009;18:956–64.
28. Floor SA, de Smet PA, et al. Documentation quality in community pharmacy: completeness of electronic patient records after patients' first visits. Ann Pharmacother. 2009;43(11): 1787–94.
29. Lau HS, Florax C, et al. The completeness of medication histories in hospital medical records of patients admitted to general internal medicine wards. Br J Clin Pharmacol. 2006;49(6): 597–603.
30. Rahimtoola H, Timmers A, et al. An evaluation of community pharmacy records in the development of pharmaceutical care in the Netherlands. Pharm World Sci. 1997;19:105–13.
31. Buurma H, De Smet PA, et al. Disease and intolerability documentation in electronic patient records. Ann Pharmacother. 2005;39:1640–6.
32. Saverno KR, Hines LE, et al. Ability of pharmacy clinical decision-support software to alert users about clinically important drug-drug interactions. J Am Med Inform Assoc. 2011;18: 32–7.
33. Hines LE, Saverno KR, et al. Pharmacists' awareness of clinical decision support in pharmacy information systems: an exploratory evaluation. Res Social Adm Pharm. 2011;7:359–68.
34. Simonaitis L, Belsito A et al. Aggregation of pharmacy dispensing data into a unified patient medication history. AMIA Annu Symp Proc. 2008;6:1135.
35. RCGP Informatics Group. Shared record professional guidance report. 2009. http://www.rcgp. org.uk/pdf/Health_Informatics_SRPG_final_report.pdf. Accessed on Feb 2012.
36. Adcock H. Electronic solution to intervention monitoring aids clinical governance. Hosp Pharm. 2006;13:137.
37. Nurgat ZA, Al-Jazairi AS, et al. Documenting clinical pharmacist intervention before and after the introduction of a web-based tool. Int J Clin Pharm. 2011;33(2):200–7.
38. Bates DW, Leape L, et al. Effect of computerised physician order entry and a team intervention on prevention of serious medication errors. J Am Med Assoc. 1998;280:1311–6.
39. Miller RA, Gardner RM, Johnson KB, Hripcsak G. Clinical decision support and electronic prescribing systems: a time for responsible thought and action. J Am Med Inform Assoc. 2005;12:403–9.
40. Farrar K. Accountability, prescribing and hospital pharmacy in an electronic, automated age. Pharm J. 1999;263:496–501.

41. Curtis C, Ford NG. Paperless electronic prescribing in a district general hospital. Pharm J. 1997;259:734–5.
42. Barker A, Kay J. Electronic prescribing improves patient safety – an audit. Hosp Pharm. 2007;14:225.
43. Slee A E-prescribing in Birmingham. Presented at the Guild of Healthcare Pharmacists/United Kingdom Clinical Pharmacy Association Information Technology Interest Group (ITIG) Seminar, Oct 2010, Birmingham. http://www.ghp.org.uk/ContentFiles/ghpitig10a.pps. Accessed on Feb 2012.

Chapter 7
Barcodes and Logistics

Introduction

Logistics – the management of the supply chain – is an essential part of any business, since the ability to supply the correct product is a pre-requisite to trade and failure to do so will lead to loss of revenue and customer dissatisfaction. While in the past, for example, following the Boots self-service case before the British High Court in 1953 [1], it has been argued that medicines are not ordinary items of commerce, they are commodities that are traded and therefore the principles of market demand and supply chain dynamics apply.

Since the development of modern IT systems, sophisticated technologies involving barcode tracking of goods and automated picking and handling have become well-established in the freight, haulage, wholesale and retail sectors but, perhaps because of the "special" nature of medicines, they are at an earlier stage of adoption in the pharmaceutical industry and pharmacy supply chain.

The pharmaceutical industry's supply chain, from manufacturer to patient, is highly fragmented and still makes little use of automatic identification and data capture techniques, such as barcodes and radio frequency product identification (RFID). As such, it can learn from the experience in leading industries (the retail, automotive and other sectors), which have transformed their supply chains reaping huge efficiency and security benefits using such automated techniques.

The availability of a seamless pharmaceutical supply chain, where electronic tracking is possible to batch or even individual pack level will provide a range of possible solutions to current issues in pharmacy and medicines management:

- Automated supply and reduction of picking errors
- Greater efficiency in the supply chain
- Authentication of medicines and prevention of counterfeit medicines
- Support for patient safety at the health service end of the supply chain
- Capability for batch recall alerts.

However, the ability to deliver these and other benefits will not be feasible without the total commitment of the industry and the government to bring about

S. Goundrey-Smith, *Information Technology in Pharmacy*,
DOI 10.1007/978-1-4471-2780-2_7, © Springer-Verlag London 2013

a harmonized and internationally agreed system. If this endeavour is not embraced, there is a high risk that other fragmented and less effective, solutions will be developed or imposed on the supply chain by politically-dominant stakeholders. This chapter will review the supply chain processes for pharmacy, the technologies that have been used in the supply chain, in particular barcode product identification, and how these technologies may be optimized to streamline the supply chain and deliver the potential benefits mentioned above.

Current Pharmaceutical Distribution Processes

Hospital and community pharmacies obtain their medicines from a number of sources. The majority are obtained through the major pharmaceutical wholesalers, although some items are obtained direct from pharmaceutical companies and a proportion of these are specials – unlicensed medicines made on an individual basis, rather than licensed medicines marketed and stockpiled on a commercial basis.

Pharmaceutical wholesalers deliver over two billion medicines each year to dispensing GP's, hospitals and community pharmacies [1], and are a major factor in the distribution of medicines in many developed countries. Wholesalers often provide a range of other marketing and merchandising support services to pharmacies they supply. As mentioned in Chap. 6, many of the community pharmacy systems in the UK were developed by the wholesalers as a free or subsidized service to pharmacies for stock control, in return for a contract to supply goods. Ethical products are normally ordered and delivered twice daily in single units, which helps to minimise stock levels.

There is an increasing trend towards "direct to purchaser" (DTP) supply schemes being introduced by large pharmaceutical manufacturers, which enables a pharmaceutical company to control the supply chain, and the end user price. Pharmaceutical companies also claim that DTP schemes are an important step towards prevention of counterfeiting, as they reduce the number of steps in the supply chain, but there is little evidence to suggest that this is the case. Pharmacists, however, are often not happy with DTP schemes because they prevent the pharmacist obtaining supplies from a single wholesaler and, in some cases, the service and delivery of these schemes has been of lower standard than from a wholesaler.

There are also issues concerning the supply of "specials". Specials are unlicensed medicines which are made to order, and there is therefore no list price for these medicines. There are however a large number of specials companies and contract manufacturers trading, so the prices of specials may be very high and there may be considerable variation in specials prices in any one healthcare economy. Also, some specials may be supplied via a wholesaler in order to enable the distribution network, and the wholesaler may add on a considerable margin, which is not visible to the end purchaser, because of the lack of a list price. The end result is that the pharmacist may be presented with a large invoice for one product, which may consist largely of profit for the specials manufacturer or the wholesaler, for which the pharmacist seeks reimbursement from the health service. With health services in all countries needing to make cost savings, there has been a move to reduce money spent on specials in the UK health service [2]. In the UK, a tariff for specials has been introduced to ensure that prices paid by pharmacies (and ultimately the NHS) are reasonable, and also to create some transparency around prices and margins in the supply chain.

At the current time, approximately 92 % of pharmaceutical drug packs have an EAN/GTIN barcode (EAN code) on the product pack (see section "Medicine Item Codes" in Chap. 1). Products that may not have an EAN code include specials, and also clinical trials medicines, hospital own manufactured items and parallel imports. The EAN code contains fixed information (Country, Company, Product and a check digit), which means it can be printed as permanent artwork on the product pack. The EAN code standard is a global, open standard, and so it ensures that a product can be identified unambiguously with no data anomalies.

Once a medicine leaves the pharmaceutical company factory gates, it may go to the patient via a number of different routes, which may not be transparent in terms of product tracking. Some products are supplied direct to pharmacies in DTP schemes, as mentioned. Some will be distributed to pharmacies via a full or short-line wholesaler. Some may be purchased from a wholesaler and then sold to a pharmacy multiple or hospital provider where they might remain in a central store or warehouse, prior to distribution to individual pharmacies in the group for dispensing. Because many products have an EAN code, the potential exists for products to be tracked through the supply chain, but this is usually not possible because not all locations will have the technology to read barcodes or software configured to store and process them. For example, while many community pharmacy systems are able to store EAN codes, very few pharmacies configure their systems to use barcodes and orders arriving from wholesalers are processed manually. This is a barrier to barcode product identification at the point of dispensing, which would have a beneficial effect on patient safety. Some pharmacies, however, use the EAN code for EPOS (Electronic Point of Sale) systems.

In the community pharmacy, the PIP code is usually used for the ordering and receipting of goods. While this code is routinely used in wholesaling in the UK, it is not machine readable so it has limited application for use with technology for medicines handling.

Procurement processes in hospital pharmacy can be manual and labour intensive. Some hospitals have implemented electronic transfer of orders and invoices, and even in these cases, the systems require manual checking. Goods are often ordered generically but supplied by brand, which can give rise to confusion.

Traditional distribution systems in hospitals are manual and are associated with a high level of ordering errors and transcription errors, which may introduce patient safety risks. Use of the EAN code enables pharmacy robots, but often this is the last point in the supply chain where electronic identifiers are used. Use of electronic ward cabinets (see Chap. 4) would improve control of the hospital pharmacy supply chain and would enable improved patient safety and tracking of medicines to ward, or even patient level, using barcode identification of medicines.

Development of Barcodes and Optical Technology

Barcodes and optical technology have been in routine use in the retail environment for product identification since the early 1970s [3]. The Universal Product Code (UPC-A) barcode first appeared in the 1970s and is still the predominant coding used in retail and logistics today. The European Article Number (EAN) 13 barcode scheme for the identification of pharmaceutical products was derived from the UPC-A schema.

However, the development of barcode schemas and their adoption has been very much driven by developments in optical imaging technology. The earliest bar code scanners were laser scanners consisting of a neon-helium filled glass tube. They were expensive to produce and therefore were not widely used. However, the advent of solid state (silicon technology) laser diodes – which was developed for use in CD and subsequently DVD players – made barcode scanners easier and cheaper to produce, and enabled barcode scanning to be more widely adopted in business and retail environments. However, the development of digital imaging technology, such as that used in document scanners, has enabled barcode methodology and use to develop further, and this will be further enabled by the development of technologies such as the digital camera array scanners, used in mobile phone cameras.

The key challenges to barcoding as the consumer industries have developed have been to make barcoding schemas hospitable to a greater number and differentiation of products, and also to store more product information for each product, to enable intelligent marketing. These challenges have certainly applied to pharmaceuticals, with an increase in the number of available pharmaceutical products over the last 30 years. Furthermore, in pharmaceuticals, while barcoding to identify products, in terms of the drug, strength, manufacturer and pack size is useful, it would be a useful development to be able to identify products to the batch level or even individual pack level, in order to handle product recall issues. However, this requires more data than can be put into a barcode using the traditional symbology. Furthermore, with smaller pack sizes and increasing regulatory requirements for packaging in certain sectors, space on the pack was at a premium. Consequently, smaller barcodes were sought after to address this issue.

Consequently, in the late 1990s a new barcode format was designed for retail use. It was called Reduced Space Symbology (RSS) and consisted of a multi-row barcode, which could be stacked, and would therefore take up less space on a pack than a UPC-A or EAN barcode, and enable more data about the product, other than product ID, to be included on the barcode. This newer barcode was renamed the GS1 barcode and is being used for some retail applications. These barcodes were designed for traditional laser barcode scanners, but each row of data needs to be scanned separately, in order to decode the whole barcode. The GS1 barcode has been used the healthcare industry in the US for some time and have been adopted to some extent by the US pharmaceutical industry to enable batch numbers and expiry dates to be carried by the barcoding, as an additional row of data.

The introduction of imaging scanners has enabled the development of two dimensional (2D) bar codes that consist of a matrix of square elements and GS1 have now adopted a 2D barcode called a data matrix code. 2D bar codes are smaller than linear barcodes, yet can code larger amounts of data. A type of 2D data matrix bar code which has originated from Japan is the QR Code, which may be used to link mobile phones with the internet to selected websites, and is being routinely used in communications, media and advertising. 2D matrix bar codes cannot be scanned by conventional laser scanners but many shops now use hand held imaging scanners, and eventually imaging scanning technology may become cheap enough to be scalable for universal retail applications. The European pharmaceutical industry is planning to adopt the 2D data matrix bar code and many companies are using data matrix codes for product tracking.

Radio Frequency Identification (RFID)

While barcode symbology systems provide an identifier through a machine-readable optical code, radio-frequency identification (RFID) systems [4] use a unique radio frequency "tag" which can be picked up by an adjacent wireless system. This means that the RFID tagged item does not need to be scanned in a directional way by a human operator, which reduces the risk of items not being tracked because they are not scanned. It also enables the use of such systems for theft prevention.

While this technology avoids the cumbersome and intrusive use of barcode scanners, which may be an advantage in the clinical environment, it is subject to the same issues that might arise with other wireless network technologies. These include (a) security of data transmission; (b) reliability of data transmission, given the geographical features of hospital buildings, and (c) collision of data with data in other wireless networks.

There may be problems due to lack of scanning due to wireless blackspots or interference of other radio frequency noise [5]. RFIDs are already used in various retail and logistics scenarios for product tracking, and while the use of RFID for identifying medicines has been discussed in the literature [5], at the current time, RFID technology is probably too expensive for widespread adoption in the healthcare sector [6]. There are also no specific standards for its use. At the current time, RFID tends to be used in some circumstances for patient tracking by health providers, whereas barcode scanning is still used for tracking medicines [7]. Use of RFIDs as identifiers for medicines would enable a more comprehensive dataset for medicines that barcodes currently allow. However, the adoption of RFID tags for medicines is not an imminent prospect, given the current slow process towards international harmonization and standardization with 2D barcodes.

The Regulatory Framework for Supply Chain Harmonisation

In 2004, the FDA published a rule that would require human prescription medicines, biological products such as vaccines and OTC medicines to have a linear bar code, which must contain the National Drug Code (NDC) number.

Use of a standard coding system (the EAN.UCC System) for pharmaceutical product identification is mandatory in Australia and in Japan for pharmaceuticals (second largest global market to the US) as well as for medical devices (both the EAN.UCC System).

In Europe, the lack of harmonisation of coding systems has led to a number of national regulators of member states to adopt proprietary coding systems that are either not workable or can only be implemented at high cost. This has happened in Belgium, Italy and Portugal.

In the UK, the Dictionary of Medicines and Devices (dm+d) will soon be the NHS standard dictionary for all medicines used in clinical messages and care records. The dm+d enables medicines to be described at the molecular level and as specific presentations and packs, so that different formulations of the same active drug can be described accurately and unambiguously. The purpose of dm+d is to underpin the NHS master files and provide the single terminology standard that will form the UK drug extension to SNOMED CT. Together these will provide the basis for electronic and human readable representation of all healthcare information, which will be contained within electronic health records (EHR) in the NHS and beyond. There is a need to map the GTIN (EAN) code to the dm+d identifier for each particular product pack (actual medicinal product pack (AMPP); this mapping would then be distributed with dm+d. This will enable continuity of medicine identification between NHS records and all points in the supply chain, which will enable greater use of technology to reduce medicine ordering, dispensing and administration errors. This change would not impinge on the usual working processes of healthcare professionals. The need for greater use of barcodes in the healthcare system in the UK, and the strategy by which this might be achieved is discussed in the 2007 report Coding for Success: Simple technology for safer patient care [8].

The European Pharmaceutical Supply Chain Working Group (EPSCWG) is an EAN International *European Healthcare Initiative* project that is aiming to establish a set of voluntary guidelines for identification, bar coding and eMessaging for the European pharmaceutical industry based upon the EAN.UCC System. These guidelines will be promoted as the 'best practice' model to regulatory bodies (e.g. European Commission, EMEA) as well as pharmaceutical companies and organisations.

A report on barcode technology [9], commissioned by the then NHS Purchasing and Supply Agency (PASA)(now the Department of Health Commercial Medicines Unit) and compiled by a cross-industry working group, strongly recommended:

• That the EAN.UCC open global standards (of product identification and RFID (EPC)) is formally selected for the coding and symbolisation for all pharmaceutical products available in the end to end (active ingredient to consumption) UK supply chain
• That a review of the general processes and practices related to scanning, relabeling and repackaging (loss of original product ID), dispensing and supply chain traceability is quickly undertaken and that the output from this review should address patient safety issues

- That a joined up work programme consisting of industry, profession and government stakeholders is established immediately to evaluate and recommend as appropriate the introduction of coding and symbolisation at all relevant levels of product packaging and processes to enable full end to end traceability, accounting for the emergence of new technologies such as RFID/EPC, defining where required migration paths to protect stakeholders' investment.

Rationale for Barcode Symbology Harmonisation

It is essential that stakeholders work together to agree an international convention for barcode identification in order to ensure a system whereby all products can be uniquely identified in the supply chain on an international basis. The danger is that one specific organization will attempt to impose its own system on the market, which is not appropriate in a market where there are many different suppliers and distributors. A proprietary system would also require the owning organisation which dictates the codes to maintain the system and to police the use of codes in the supply chain. This is beyond the remit of individual pharmaceutical manufacturers or healthcare providers. It also might encourage the growth of more coding that is specific to the pharmaceutical sector, and lead to further fragmentation of coding data. There is also a greater risk of overlap between systems used by different suppliers in different sectors and different countries, which would compromise the use of coding for unique product identification. Also, proprietary identifiers are not interoperable with other identifiers and cannot be communicated with non-compatible systems.

However, an international standardized coding structure enables requirements (requisitions, orders, delivery notes, invoices) to be communicated in a common language and identification of medicines according to a common format. This will enable true international interoperability and the potential for international e-commerce. The way to achieve this is through a global open standard code structure, which provides the detailed structure to support medicine identification, but is compatible and continuous with other areas of trade and commerce. EAN coding offers the appropriate features for an international coding standard for pharmaceuticals:

- The code structure and actual code numbers are controlled by central organisations. Without central control, there is no guarantee that codes are unique and immediately recognizable.
- Widely-used linear symbology, which is the most widely used anywhere in the world.
- Code structure is numeric and nonsignificant, and therefore can apply to any industry.
- EAN coding is present in many different sectors in the manufacture, retail and healthcare.
- EAN codes may be used with many types of data carrier: bar code, RSS, RFID depending on application.

The aspiration of a <u>seamless pharmaceutical supply chain</u> with electronic management and tracking will not be achieved without a concerted effort to develop standards and harmonization of supply chain coding and processes across the industry. This will involve all stakeholders, such as:

- Patients
- Clinicians
- Pharmacy Multiple HQs
- Pharmaceutical Manufacturers
- Wholesalers
- Parallel Importers
- Retailers
- Community pharmacies
- Hospital pharmacies
- Logistics and transportation
- Trade associations
- Government and associated agencies

The problem with the international barcode harmonization initiative is that the process is slow [4] and there is the danger that optical barcode technology will have been superseded operationally by the time any international standard has been achieved, and that there will be no coherent standardisation strategy for RFID tagging.

Benefits of Barcode and Optical Technology in Pharmacy and Medicines Management

<u>Barcode technology</u> has the potential to improve the efficiency of the supply chain and to improve the accuracy of product identification at each point in the supply chain.

Patient Safety

As has already been discussed, there is a clear need to improve patient safety, particularly in the processes of the prescribing, supply and administration of medicines.

The <u>Audit Commission's Spoonful of Sugar report</u> [5] indicated that in an average UK hospital, there are:

- 7,000 drug administrations per day
- The rate of <u>medicine administration errors</u> is on average 5 % (varies between 3 and 10 %)
- 350 errors per day relating to medicines administration
- Some of these cause adverse drug events (ADEs), which increase the length of stay in hospital by on average 8.5 days [10]
- 1 in 1,000 of all medicines administration errors is potentially fatal.

Bates et al. [11] identified the following medication error rates:

- Prescribing – 56 %
- Administration – 34 %
- Transcription – 6 %
- Dispensing – 4 %

There are a number of general principles that relate to risk management in the medication use process.

(a) Human error, or operator error, where the process is being facilitated by electronic systems, is a major risk element in medicines management, since, at various points in the medicines use process, human actions and decisions are required. The potential for human error increases when tasks are repetitive or inherently boring. The use of automated systems, such as EP systems, pharmacy robots and automated ward cabinets, therefore reduces risks with medicine selection and stock control processes that are repetitive, iterative or which are complex, but predictable.

(b) Medication errors are often multi-factorial in their causation. To give a simplistic example: a patient is prescribed Amitriptyline 10 mg tablets, and the directions are 1–2 at night. The hyphen on the drug chart becomes illegible, and the patient is given 12 (12) amitriptyline 10 mg tablets in error. In this situation, there are three potential factors which gave rise to this incident. Firstly, the prescriber's instructions were not completely unambiguous; secondly, the pharmacist did not clarify the directions and, thirdly, the nurse administered the dose without querying it. Situations of this nature commonly arise in busy clinical environments and the likelihood of such errors increases with workload, if systems are not in place to monitor the medicines management process. Furthermore, if just one of these factors had been addressed, the incident would not have happened. This phenomenon has been described in medicines risk studies as the so-called "Swiss cheese effect" [12] – i.e. the skewer can pass right through the middle of the cheese, if all the holes line up. Furthermore, at a statistical level, a number of different types of error may contribute to the overall medication error rate in a hospital. These are the sort of statistics that are assessed in quantitative studies of EP systems and other automated systems.

(c) As a general rule, the incidence of medication errors may be reduced by having standard operating procedures (SOPs) in place, which anticipate likely causes of errors, and which reduce any variations in working practice arising from exceptional circumstances. These should closely reflect, and aim to standardise, normative working practice. Each step may be straightforward and even self-explanatory, but documentation of the procedure helps members of staff to follow it, so that it becomes instinctive for them. An example of this is the checking of a patient's hospital number as well as their name, prior to administering drugs.

Patient safety is a key political issue for the UK Government (as well as the European Commission). Authoritative reports such as 'A Spoonful of Sugar' [13] and 'Organisation with a Memory' [10] have underlined the extent of medication errors – that approximately 60 patients die each day due to adverse drug errors. Furthermore, as reports in both the UK [14] and the US [10] have indicated, the knock-on costs of a high patient risk environment leads to significant costs in additional hospital stays plus clinical negligence claims.

An automated supply chain and the use of bar codes to enable automated product identification and picking, has the potential to improve patient safety.

Many of the medication errors occur as a result of a lack of machine-readable codes, which significantly increases the risk of human visual identification errors (Many packs are of similar name, size and appearance). An automated supply chain and the use of bar codes to enable automated product identification and picking, has the potential to improve patient safety.

The certainty of identification of pharmaceutical products enabled by scanning will reduce medication errors by the elimination of error-prone manual processes thereby saving peoples' lives. Linkage of accurate product information to the patient's electronic health record (EHR) will deliver even greater safety benefits – ensuring the right product, to the right patient, at the right dose, at the right time, by the right route.

Security of the Supply Chain

Product security is a key requirement in the management of the pharmaceutical supply chain. Theft from the supply chain, either directly or by fraudulent activity, is costly to the industry. Furthermore, the risk of counterfeit medicines is a key issue for the pharmaceutical industry and its reputation, as counterfeit medicines are detrimental both to patient safety and the product brand. Furthermore, counterfeit medicines may enter the UK supply chain through unusual routes, which may not be easily detectable.

The development of batch/serial traceability through bar codes and RFID has the potential to prevent theft from the supply chain, to determine the routes by which illicit products may be entering the supply chain, and to identify counterfeit products.

Tracking of Supply Chain Efficiency

Accurate product tracking within the supply chain using either optical barcode technology or RFID allows transparency and traceability within the supply chain. With scanning points along the supply chain, and a standard coding system, all transactional processes – ordering, invoicing, availability enquiries, returns, owings – could be logged and audited. The supply chain could then be actively managed to improve efficiency. This would enable a move towards smaller stock surplus, "just in time" stock management and shorter replenishment lead times. This would reduce capital tied up in stock, reduce administration costs and reduce inventory costs, with considerable savings across the supply chains. Analysis of other supply chains, such as fast-moving consumer goods, has shown that considerable cost savings can be achieved using electronic technologies to monitor and manage the supply chain. Product tracking within the supply chain also provides the potential for:

- Automated product recall
- Contract and performance monitoring
- Operation of commercial and buying schemes by pharmaceutical manufacturers and wholesalers

Currently, it is not possible to track products through the supply chain, because barcode scanning is not enabled at all points in the supply chain.

Intraoperability

More health economies are using a range of technologies for medicines management, such as electronic ordering, electronic prescribing and clinician workflow, pharmacy robots and electronic ward cabinets, as well as the pharmacy system. As has been mentioned previously, there is a need for interfaces between all of these systems, and the development of appropriate interfaces to allow true intraoperability between systems is not straightforward, often because these systems are using different internal coding systems. GTIN/EAN codes provide a international standard for product identification, and therefore the availability of EAN codes as the standard system for identifying medicines, and their active use within pharmacy and e-prescribing technologies, will promote intraoperability and integrated use of all of the systems and technologies described in this book. Standardised product coding, data structures and data carriers will ensure interoperability throughout the supply chain as well as within clinical and pharmacy IT systems.

Furthermore, mapping of EAN codes to the dm ± d will close the gap between the identification of medicines in electronic health records (EHRs) and NHS IT systems and services, and the identification of medicines at any point in the supply chain, right up to the patient's bedside. This provides a much larger framework of intraoperability between different IT systems than use of EAN codes alone.

E-Commerce in Pharmacy

There is growing use of e-ordering and e-commerce in the pharmacy sector. While community pharmacies have been placing orders electronically through their pharmacy systems, via modem or e-fax, for some years, they have not had an automated means of processing the goods received and invoices, which has implications for stock control, especially in larger pharmacies. Furthermore, the ordering process for hospital pharmacies has been traditionally paper-based – with generation of paper orders, based on product usage data, faxing of the orders with postal confirmation, and then manual processing of goods received, and invoices sent to the finance department for payment.

The universal availability of machine-readable codes for medicines, together with electronic signatures/authorisation, brings with it the possibility of electronic ordering. There have been a variety of approaches to electronic ordering, from standard <u>electronic data interchange (EDI)</u> via a modem link, <u>XML terminology</u>, transmission of order data via an Excel file or use of standard messaging formats, such as the <u>pharmacy messaging service (PMS)</u>, which was developed for NHS purchasing in the UK.

Electronic ordering offers the following benefits:

- Reduction in number of <u>ordering errors</u>. The figure quoted from a study by DH CMU (NHS PASA) in the UK is that, if 90 % of orders are placed electronically, there will only be 5 % of ordering errors or exceptions.
- Reduction in the cost of <u>procurement administration</u>
- More streamlined procurement processes and improved timeliness of order transmission
- Greater transparency of the order process and ease of monitoring
- The order items can be more easily matched to the invoiced items, to monitor order fulfilment and ensure accurate payments.

A number of wholesalers have developed electronic ordering systems, such as Medecator from AAH Pharmaceuticals. In the UK, the Luton and Dunstable Hospital installed the Windows-based Powergate e-commerce system [15], which enabled the mapping of products from the pharmacy system to the supplier's/wholesaler's electronic catalogue(s), usually using the <u>EAN code</u>, and ensured that electronic orders could be sent from the <u>pharmacy system</u>, and be fully readable by the supplier computer system. The order would then be fulfilled and delivered with a concomitant electronic invoice, which would enable electronic booking in of goods on the pharmacy system, and also electronic transfer of invoice data to the finance department. The e-ordering system enabled the department to improve stock profiling, develop saving strategies for high-cost lines and released 10 h' staff time from the purchasing process each week. The system also had a beneficial effect on relationships with wholesalers.

At the Greater Glasgow & Clyde NHS Board in Scotland, <u>pharmacy automation</u> was used together with electronic trading (wherever possible) to enable centralised procurement and distribution to hospital wards and departments across the region [16]. The centralisation of procurement led to some concerns from suppliers about the visibility of the <u>supply chain</u> beyond the procurement hub. However, these concerns were addressed with appropriate information feeds from individual hospital sites, and building up good relationships with wholesaler/supplier managers.

Reduction of Dispensing Errors

It is recognized that <u>barcode scanning</u> during the dispensing process has the potential to reduce <u>dispensing errors</u> [17]. This may be done either in conjunction with a pharmacy robot or as a stand-alone process with a barcode scanner linked to the pharmacy system. Nevertheless, there are various barriers to implementation of barcode scanning for medicines verification in the dispensing process, especially if it is a stand-alone process relying on manual scanning by a member of staff.

These include:

- Interruption of the usual pharmacy workflow.
- Availability of the technology (many community pharmacy systems are not configured to use barcodes at the point of dispensing).
- Staff training and engagement on the benefits of using a barcode scanning system.

Automated systems have the potential to reduce errors and manage risk at the supply end of the medicines use process. The UK Audit Commission's "Spoonful of Sugar" report [18], published in 2001, highlighted the potential of pharmacy automation to reduce dispensing error rates. Following on from that report, many hospital pharmacy departments constructed business cases to install automated dispensing systems (pharmacy robots), and to re-engineer pharmacy services. The operational aspects of these, and their relationship with EP systems, have been discussed in the previous chapter. A further study by Beard and Candlish at Sunderland [10] examined the extent to which an EP system could reduce the incidence of dispensing errors. An important general factor is that, because traditional dispensing is a manual process, error rates will to some extent be dependent on the number of staff present in a dispensary, and so dispensing error figures should be adjusted to take this into account, and be expressed as errors per member of staff. The authors found that the use of the EP system for inpatient medicine ordering led to an dispensing error rate of 0.0029 errors per person, compared to 0.0045–0.0057 errors per person in other areas of the hospital. One of the pharmacies in the Trust used barcode product selection, which achieved a slightly lower dispensing error rate of 0.0022 errors per person. Due to the high ratio of staff to prescriptions, and the highly controlled environment, the lowest dispensing error rate was in the Trust's chemotherapy manufacturing facility, where the authors calculated an error rate of zero.

Electronic Medicines Administration

As discussed in Chap. 3, BCMA has the potential to reduce a significant proportion of medication errors relating to the administration of medicines. Furthermore, in conjunction with pharmacy robotics, barcodes can facilitate an end-to-end (closed loop) safe medication system [19]. Barcode technology has also been used by EP systems in order to reduce errors in the medication administration process on the ward. The patient's wristband barcode is scanned prior to a medicine administration event to confirm patient identity, and the barcode on the medicine is scanned to confirm the identity of the medicine to be administered. Medicines administration with the assistance of barcodes to identify either the patient or the drug may contribute to reductions in levels of medicine administration errors at the point of administration.

The EP implementation at Charing Cross Hospital, London, UK [20], used barcode identification of patients. At each medicine administration event, the EP system required the patient's barcode to be scanned, in order for the patient's drawer on the electronic drug trolley to be released, so that the nurse could access the patient's medication. This barcode patient identification function caused the percentage of occasions where the patient identity was not checked to be reduced from 82.6 to 18.9 %. However, system compliance was limited by practices such as sticking the patient's barcode to their bedside cupboard, rather than to their wristband.

Poon et al. [21] conducted a study of 115,164 medicines administration events before implementation of barcode medicine administration, and 253,984 administration events after implementation. They found that target adverse events were reduced by 74 % and all adverse events were reduced by 63 %, and that the greater the proportion of doses scanned, the higher the error reduction rates possible. Nolen et al. [22] studied the use of barcode medicine administration (BCMA) in anaesthetics for cardiac surgery cases (n = 870). They found that the BCMA process increased the available information on peri-operative drug administration by 21.7 %, and the availability of drug cost data by 18.8 %. Furthermore, the time required to process the operating room anaesthesia record was reduced by 8 min per case, following full implementation of the system.

Miller et al. [23] has indicated that BCMA can reduce medication errors and improve patient safety. However, because the process of medicines administration by barcode scanning is potentially interruptive, there are various work-arounds (BCMA work-arounds) that nurses and pharmacists may use to bypass the system. In a study of five hospitals, Koppel et al. [24] have studied BCMA work-arounds and identified 15 work-arounds, with 31 causes of different types. Reasons for work-arounds [25] include:

- Inability to scan medicines because a scanner is not available at the point of medicines administration
- Lack of awareness of the hospital's BCMA process (bank/agency staff, but also new staff and staff who are not usually involved with medicines administration)
- Shortage of time
- Delay in computer response
- Administration of a medicine prior to prescribing

McNulty et al. [26] discussed strategies for dealing with the problem of BCMA work-around. These include:

(a) encouraging a better culture of ownership of the system among nursing staff
(b) improving the infrastructure to address known technical issues (e.g. wireless black spots)
(c) an effective staff training programme, and better engagement of staff during the implementation period.
(d) greater use of "hard stops" in the system (i.e. ensuring that a medicine is not available for administration without following the procedure – e.g.

linking BCMA to electronic ward cabinets). However, hard stops may be highly disruptive and implementers should consider the unintended consequences in each scenario.

The culture of ownership of the system is important and, while BCMA has the potential to resolve many medication errors at the point of administration, managers should remember that different staff groups with have different priorities with BCMA implementation [27]. Pharmacy staff will want to ensure that the stock and inventory is controlled, whereas nursing staff will want to ensure that the system is usable at the point of medicine administration.

There are potential barriers to the use of barcodes for medicine identification at the point of administration:

1. It is recognised that a proportion of medicinal products do not have barcodes [28]. This is especially the case with "specials", parallel imports and some hospital manufactured products. There would need to an increase in the proportion of medicines that could be accurately identified by barcode for barcode medicine identification to be feasible in a variety of secondary care specialities.
2. Barcode medicine identification relies on original barcoded packs being used for medicine administration at ward level. While this may be the norm in some countries, it is not routinely the case in the UK.
3. Barcode medicine identification on wards relies on the availability, configuration and scalability of the appropriate hardware

In the long term, the use of barcodes may also be limited by harmonisation issues and obsolescence, due to development of RFID (radio frequency identification) technology [4].

The benefits of improved operational efficiency, together with patient safety features, drive additional economic benefits. These include reduction in reworking and reordering, improved product availability, reduction in waste (expired medicines), reduced compensation claims, lower litigation costs and better bed/patient throughput (less bed days lost due to adverse events).

Pharmacy Workflow Tracking

As well as tracking of medicines through the supply chain, barcodes can also be used to track prescriptions through the pharmacy dispensing process (pharmacy tracking). In smaller pharmacies, this may not be necessary, but workflow tracking is useful in large hospital pharmacy departments, where there may be a large workload with prescriptions and orders arriving in the department from various different locations.

As previously discussed in Chap. 3, the efficiency of the discharge process in hospitals is important to ensure good bed management, allocation of resources and continuity of care. However, the process of dispensing discharge prescriptions or TTOs (to take out medicines) is one that often causes problems for hospital pharmacy. The discharge prescription is initiated on the ward after the medical team has decided that a patient can be discharged and is sent to the pharmacy to be prepared. The discharge prescription may genuinely take some time to prepare if it contains a large number of medicines, or specialist items. However, there are many other factors that can affect the time it takes for the discharge medication to be prepared. The junior doctor may not immediately write the discharge prescription when the consultant tells the patient they can go home. The preparation of the discharge prescription may be delayed while the nursing staff arrange transport for the patient. There may be a delay in the discharge prescription leaving the ward, depending on other ward staff activities. The discharge prescription may travel to the pharmacy by a circuitous route, because of portering schedules. However, this means that pharmacy managers often receive a great number of complaints about discharge prescriptions that have not been done on time, when not all of the delays are due to the pharmacy department.

Some of the problems can be obviated by introducing electronic prescribing, where the discharge prescription is generated electronically on the ward and transferred automatically to a pharmacy workstation for checking and dispensing, and by the use of pharmacy robots to speed up the picking process. However, some pharmacies have introduced workload tracking using barcode scanning, to monitor the physical throughput of the dispensing process.

The prescription or order is assigned a barcode when it is received into the pharmacy department. It is the scanned using a fixed or wireless scanner at various points in its journey through the pharmacy department:

- When the clinical checks are made
- When it is labeled
- When the items are picked for dispensing
- When the final check is made
- When the completed prescription leaves the pharmacy

A picture can then be built up of the working patterns and throughput of the pharmacy department, and reports can be generated of, for example, the percentage of discharge prescriptions completed within 2 h. Some systems have included tracking points on wards as well, so that the journey of the prescription from and to the ward can also be monitored.

This enables pharmacy managers to differentiate between genuine complaints, where the pharmacy team could take actions to improve the service, and situations that have arisen through factors beyond the control of the pharmacy department. This enables resolution of disputes with wards and departments, and also identifies areas of weakness in the pharmacy processes and workflow bottlenecks, where service improvements could be made.

As with other systems that change the usual working practices of the department, staff engagement and ownership of the system is vital if it is to be used effectively for all prescriptions, and meaningful data gathered. Introduction of these systems may be viewed with some suspicion by pharmacy staff, who may feel that their work is being scrutinized, and that they are being subjected to criticism. However, staff will see the benefits if the system is being used to provide evidence of their hard work, and to prevent the pharmacy department being treated unfairly by clinicians and ward staff.

As well as pharmacy tracking, barcode and RFID tagging systems would also have applications as asset tracking systems for pharmacies, to track the use of hardware and equipment, such as computers, printers, hand-held devices and other electrical equipment. This will ensure the security of equipment and can be used to monitor the lifecycle of the equipment (e.g. servicing and decommissioning dates) and scheduling routine maintenance (e.g. portable appliance testing (PAT) schedules). Asset tracking applications would be useful for monitoring the location and use of hardware from which patient records can be accessed, in order to meet information governance requirements.

Conclusion

The use of a barcodes and other symbologies are essential to ensure that the majority of medicine packs have a machine-readable identifier, so that they can be identified clearly and unambiguously by automated systems. However, there is a challenge in coordinating and harmonising medicine coding systems internationally to ensure that universal product identification is possible, thereby ensuring international e-business initiatives with pharmaceuticals. There is also a need to ensure that various systems are configured to read medicine codes at different points across the supply chain as this will enable e-commerce, supply chain tracking and efficiency and patient safety at the point of dispensing and medicine administration. There is also a need to map medicine item codes with dm + d codes to ensure that there is a link between systems for the supply of medicines and records of the clinical use of medicines. Barcodes may also have applications for tracking prescriptions within pharmacies.

References

1. Anderson S. Making medicines: a brief history of pharmacy and pharmaceuticals. London: Pharmaceutical Press; 2005. p. 127.
2. British Association of Pharmaceutical Wholesalers. http://www.bapw.net/about-pharmaceutical-wholesaling. Accessed on 2012.
3. Goundrey-Smith SJ, Hopkins R. Specials are important and here to stay. Pharm J. 2011;287:287.
4. Cross-Industry Working Group. Underpinning patient safety: recommendations and Guidance for product coding within the UK pharmaceutical supply chain. 2004. http://cmu.dh.gov.uk/. Accessed on Sep 2012.
5. Adcock H. RFID raises issues associated with privacy and data collision. Hosp Pharm. 2006;13:138.
6. Lahtela A, Saranto K. RFID and medication care. Stud Health Technol Inform. 2009;146:747–8.
7. Kumar S, Swanson E, et al. RFID in the healthcare supply chain: usage and application. Int J Health Care Qual Assur. 2009;22:67–81.
8. Lahtela A, Hassinen M. Requirements for radio frequency identification in healthcare. Stud Health Technol Inform. 2009;150:720–4.

 9. Department of Health (UK). Coding for success – simple technology for safer patient care. 2007. http://www.dh.gov.uk/en/Publicationsandstatistics/Publications/PublicationsPolicyAndGuidance/DH_066082. Accessed on Mar 2012.
10. Audit Commission. A spoonful of sugar – medicines management in NHS Hospitals. London: Audit Commission; 2001.
11. Vincent C, Neale G. Adverse events in British hospitals: preliminary retrospective record review. Br Med J. 2001;322:517–9.
12. Bates DW, Leape L, et al. Effect of computerised physician order entry and a team intervention on prevention of serious medication errors. J Am Med Assoc. 1998;280:1311–6.
13. Reason J. Human error: models and management. Br Med J. 2000;320:768–70.
14. Department of Health (UK). An organisation with a memory. 2000. http://www.dh.gov.uk/en/Publicationsandstatistics/Publications/PublicationsPolicyAndGuidance/DH_4065083.
15. Kohn LT, Corrigan JM, Donaldson MD, editors. To err is human: building a safer health system. Washington, D.C.: National Academy Press; 1999.
16. Palmer D. Procuring medicines – principles & practice of e-commerce. Hosp Pharm. 2006;13:402–3.
17. Lanningan N. Centralised procurement and distribution of medicines in a large NHS Board in Scotland – the possible model for the future? Br J Med Procurement. 2010;2(1):8–12.
18. Nanji KC, Cina J, et al. Overcoming barriers to the implementation of a pharmacy bar code scanning system for medication dispensing: a case study. J Am Med Inform Assoc. 2009;16: 645–50.
19. Beard R, Candlish C. Is electronic prescribing the best system for preventing pharmacy dispensing errors. Br J Healthc Comput. 2007;24:15–8.
20. Bepko RJ, Moore JR, et al. Implementation of a pharmacy automation system (robotics) to ensure patient medication safety at Norwalk Hospital. Qual Manag Health Care. 2009;18: 103–14.
21. Franklin BD, O'Grady K, et al. The impact of a closed-loop electronic prescribing and administration system on prescribing errors, administration errors and staff time: a before and after study. Qual Saf Health Care. 2007;16:279–84.
22. Poon EG, Cina JL, et al. Medication dispensing errors and potential adverse drug events before and after implementing bar code technology in the pharmacy. Ann Intern Med. 2006;145: 426–34.
23. Nolen AL, Rodes 2nd WD. Bar-code medication administration system for anesthetics: effects on documentation and billing. Am J Health Syst Pharm. 2008;65:655–9.
24. Miller DF, Fortier CR, et al. Barcode medication administration technology: characterisation of high-alert medication triggers and clinician workarounds. Ann Pharmacother. 2011;Feb:1.
25. Koppel R, Wetterneck T, et al. Workarounds to barcode medication administration systems: their occurrences, causes and threats to patient safety. J Am Med Inform Assoc. 2008;15: 408–23.
26. Van Onzenoort HA, Van den Plas A, et al. Factors influencing bar-code verification by nurses during medication administration in a Dutch hospital. Am J Health Syst Pharm. 2008;65: 644–8.
27. McNulty J, Donelly E, et al. Methodologies for sustaining barcode medication administration compliance. A multi-disciplinary approach. J Healthc Inf Manag. 2009;23:30–3.
28. Agrawal A, Glasser AR. Barcode medication. Administration implementation in an acute care hospital and lessons learned. J Healthc Inf Manag. 2009;23(4):24–9.

Chapter 8
Future Prospects in Pharmacy IT

While there is now experience of discrete IT systems in medicines management – pharmacy/stock control, prescribing, decision support, electronic health records and supply automation – the use of IT to provide an integrated pharmacy and medicines management service has not yet been fully realised. This has been for a number of reasons:

- Technical barriers to intraoperability – lack of effective interfaces, networking, common server infrastructure or communications technology
- Project and change management inertia within the organisation
- Lack of political will within health services and providers to implement enterprise-wide solutions
- Unwillingness of software suppliers to work together to develop integrated solutions because of commercial or intellectual property (IP) ownership considerations.

However, the greatest benefits will be realised in terms of patient safety, improved quality of care and workflow efficiencies and best use of resources, when systems can be used together in an integrated manner to support best practice in medicine, and organisational objectives.

This chapter will explore some of the future technologies that could be used in prescribing and pharmacy and which might enable end-to-end medicines management. Some of the sociopolitical aspects of IT adoption which might affect technology adoption – for example, professional engagement, development of professional standards and clinical IT education and training will also be explored.

Towards Integrated IT Systems in Pharmacy Practice

As has been discussed in previous chapters, the interfacing of pharmacy and prescribing IT applications with other systems, such as patient administration systems (PAS), pathology systems, and specialist clinical applications – is desirable in order to provide improved quality of care and patient safety within the organisation and

S. Goundrey-Smith, *Information Technology in Pharmacy*,
DOI 10.1007/978-1-4471-2780-2_8, © Springer-Verlag London 2013

a seamless workflow for the healthcare professional. As discussed, a seamless workflow promotes organisational efficiency and reduces risks associated with the rekeying of prescription data or the prescription data not being available to all users in real time. Therefore, a pharmacy or electronic prescribing system should draw its patient demographic data from the PAS, take a feed from the pathology system for test results and then transmit any medicine orders placed directly to the pharmacy system, which may also have an ongoing interface with a pharmacy robot. The interfaces described above are established requirements for pharmacy and electronic prescribing systems and have been delivered in various different ways in different installations and with different products. However, an area as yet to be fully explored is that of interfaces or integration with other devices – for example, mobile phones, diagnostic monitoring devices, electronic intravenous pumps ("smart" pumps) etc. Interfaces, or integration, with these and other devices will enable a wider range of IT support for medicines management – e.g. electronic prescribing in conjunction with telecare/telemedicine, or remote monitoring of medicines given by the intravenous route in critical care facilities.

The terms *interface* and *integration* are both used here, but they are not synonymous. In this context, *interface* is used to describe a data link between two stand-alone software applications, to enable the intraoperability of the two applications. *Integration* describes how a device, which may have limited operating software of its own, is linked into another system, which not only channels data to and from the device, but also provides the software routines to control and drive the device. The device thus becomes a integral part of the bigger system.

The point of interface or integration may be upstream from the prescribing workflow – monitoring devices, especially in the intensive care unit scenario – or downstream from the prescribing workflow – devices to facilitate therapy or drug delivery.

Device integration upstream of the prescribing process generally has as its goal the facilitation of clinical decision support. It is recognised that decision support tools are an essential aspect of any system which handles information about prescribing and medicines [1], and that decision support applications have been in use in the United States to support prescribing well before the widespread introduction of computerised ordering of medicines (CPOE) [2]. However, as discussed in Chap. 1, decision support tools require accurate input information, in order to give an appropriate clinical warning to the user. Many decision support functionalities for medicines – for example, drug interactions, duplicate therapy and drug doubling checking – are internally referential, as they use data that are already within the drug database of an EP system; data that are relatively static. Other decision support functions – such as sensitivity checking, contraindications and drug-disease warnings – rely on data from systems that are external to the system, usually on the PAS – such as patient diagnosis or concomitant conditions. These functions are more problematic because, although these data too are relatively static, there are potential issues with the currency of the patient-related data on a PAS record, with the effective transmission of that data between the PAS and the pharmacy or prescribing system, and with conflict between data values stored in two different locations.

For example, an electronic prescribing (EP) system may have links with a pathology system, so that clinicians can review test results prior to prescribing drugs, or amending drug doses. Electronic access to pathology system test ordering and results review functionality, along with EP functions, as part of an integrated clinical workstation is already a reality for some healthcare providers. However, it is to be hoped that in future there would be a direct data pull from a pathology system to an EP system in order to facilitate the prescribing of certain drugs. For example, whenever a diuretic is prescribed, the system will automatically retrieve the latest potassium result from the pathology system, and display it (together with the date that the sample was taken) on the prescribing screen. There could also be the option for the prescriber to order new pathology tests from the prescribing screen. As well as specific monitoring tests for individual drugs (for example, electrolytes with diuretics, or haematology results (haemoglobin, serum iron etc.) for anaemia treatments), there is the possibility of a batch feed of antibiotic susceptibilities to support a more complex decision support module for antibiotic prescribing. Also, it is to be hoped that, eventually, hardware advances (monitor resolution enhancements) will allow oncologists prescribing chemotherapy and adjuvant agents on an EP system to access the radiology system functions and PACS on the same workstation.

However, while the integrations described above can improve the prescribing decision support process, the logical goal of clinical decision support in electronic prescribing is a system that provides decision support intuitively, working with dynamic data from patient monitoring devices, such as blood pressure and blood gas monitoring devices.

In general terms, the EP software would respond to variations in dynamic monitoring data – for example, threshold or out-of-range triggers – and send a warning to the clinician, either on screen on the application, or routed via a pager or SMS text message, advising them of the therapeutic options for the patient. In some care situations, especially critical care scenarios where the EP system was linked downstream to a syringe driver, it would be reasonable – and indeed necessary – for the EP system to make automatic dose adjustments, based on monitoring results.

Smart Pumps

Device integration downstream of the prescribing process is generally concerned with the automated scheduling and delivery of treatment to the patient. One example of this is the integration of a syringe driver with an EP system. Syringe drivers are devices that deliver injectable medicines from a syringe at a set rate of infusion. The device is programmable with the required infusion rate, and can detect blockages in the line and other interruptions to the flow rate. Syringe drivers with highly sophisticated control mechanisms are often referred to in the literature as "smart" pumps. These devices therefore have the potential to reduce human errors associated with the administration of intravenous medicines. However, it has been determined [3] that smart pump technology alone is unlikely to reduce medication errors without:

(a) interface with an EP system, or an electronic patient record (EPR) system
(b) barcode based medicines administration functionality
(c) pharmacy information systems

Integration of a syringe pump with an EP system would enable, for example, a patient on a intensive care unit to be given a continuous infusion of isosorbide dinitrate injection in a Graseby type syringe driver, driven by an EP system. When the patient's heart rate changed, a warning message would be sent to a prescriber. The prescriber would adjust the infusion rate on the electronic administration profile of the EP system (possibly remotely), and the infusion rate would be automatically changed on the syringe driver.

Oncology Systems

Another area where there is established experience of integration of systems dealing with prescribing and pharmacy with medical devices is in the field of oncology systems. Cancer treatment protocols are increasingly mixed-modality in their format; that is to say that a particular protocol for the treatment of a certain type of cancer might consist in total of some cycles of chemotherapy and some cycles of radiotherapy. Thus, in recent years, there has been an increasing need for oncology clinic management systems to be interfaced with radiotherapy treatment equipment, so that the clinic management software can schedule and deliver radiotherapy treatment as well as chemotherapy treatments. There are therefore a number of oncology systems that offer interfaces and integration with radiotherapy treatment machines. In some of these cases, clinic management software is developed as an add-on to the device control software, and this may not be satisfactory for providing full oncology prescribing functionality. In other cases, device integration is provided as part of a comprehensive suite of oncology clinic software. However, in either case, the fact remains that radiotherapy device integration expertise has been gained specifically within oncology management software and it may not be easy for software vendors to develop radiotherapy device integration within the context of a comprehensive general EP solution.

Challenges of Device Integration

Device integration, however, presents a number of major challenges to the advanced development of EP systems:

(a) The ability of EP software vendors to keep up with developments in medical device technology and produce appropriate interface and control routines for the devices that are in current use.
(b) The use of appropriate system algorithms for device control and data feeds.
(c) The development of appropriate data standards to support intraoperability between different device types.

Various larger <u>software vendors</u> have conducted some work on device integration but many of the interfaces and software routines developed are only at the prototype stage. The universal clinical use of a range of device interfaces in hospitals and healthcare provider organisations is still very much in the future, with the exception of centres where there is in-house healthcare informatics expertise, and a proven record of healthcare IT innovation.

Smart Packaging

Medicine adherence, or <u>compliance</u>, is a problem for healthcare professionals, carers, the health service – and ultimately, for patients, who do not receive the treatment they have been prescribed. It has been estimated that between 20 and 50 % of patients are not adherent to their medication [4]. Furthermore, a recent systematic review of medicines management in the UK suggests that only 4–21 % of patients are receiving the optimum benefit of their medication [5], and adherence is an important factor in this.

The reasons for non-adherence are many and various. They include:

- The patient simply forgetting to take their medication.
- Off-putting side effects of the medication.
- Lack of tangible efficacy of the medication.
- Greater than once daily frequency of administration [6].
- Inability to understand complex dosing instructions.
- The patient exercising their prerogative of choice for a variety of personal or social reasons.

Regardless of the reason for non-adherence, the end results are the same – patients who suffer adverse effects because they are not taking a prescribed medicine (especially if they are admitted to hospital and then given the medicine in a supervised manner), and excessive amounts of wasted medicine. The cost of non-adherence, however, is much more than the cost of not taking the medicine – it encompasses the cost of the disease not being treated, in terms of working days lost and reduction in quality of life, with associated acute treatment and hospital admission costs. Technologies are now available that enable adherence monitoring for patients taking medicines for long-term, chronic conditions which, if implemented, would not only improve adherence, but would have far-reaching implications for pharmacy practice. One such technology is the <u>"smart" pack</u>, where a medicine blister pack has a microchip incorporated into it, to enable the capture of <u>medicines usage data</u>. Such a device will:

- Record when a medicine is taken or administered.
- Record responses to simple monitoring questions following each dose (after taking the tablet from the pack the patient is prompted to respond ("Is your blood sugar normal?" (Yes/No) or "How do you feel?" (Lickert scale response)).

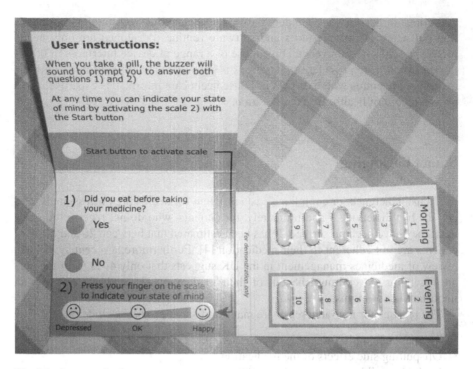

Fig. 8.1 Smart packaging

- Give a reminder for next dose (pack bleeps at required time)
- Provide other features such as expiry date warning, storage conditions monitoring and tamper alerts.

Data from these devices could be downloaded to a mobile phone or other reading software to build up a record of individual patient adherence data, which could be used as a prompt for patient counselling by healthcare professionals.

Given the widespread use of blister packaging for solid dose forms, this type of technology has the potential to become commonplace once device manufacturing costs decrease and technical standards are available to support them.

A number of electronic devices have been developed to deal with medicines adherence. These include the Aardex MEMS device, which has been trialled extensively in the UK. This device will record when the cap is removed for a patient to take a dose. However, this does not necessarily correlate to the patient taking a tablet and this is, of course, the limiting factor with this device.

"Smart packs", where a blister pack has a microchip to record information about the use of the medicine, as outlined above, have previously been prototyped by Cypak (Fig. 8.1), and Stora Enso. Cypak and Stora Enso produce intelligent blister packs, which enable compliance data gathering, as described above.

However, while the technology exists to monitor medicines adherence using such electronic devices, there is a need for a data standard to enable the storage and communication of data generated by these devices. Lack of standard datasets has in the past been identified as a major factor for the lack of widespread interface between medical devices and electronic prescribing systems [7]. However, a data standard – IEEE 11072–10472 – has now been developed to support data collection by medicines adherence devices. This world data standard is an open standard, which allows any device manufacturer to join and adopt the standard. This means that:

- The dataset can be adopted to enable electronic medicines adherence data collection in a variety of treatment presentations – for example, injectables and inhalers as well as blister packs.
- The adoption of the standard is not adversely affected by major changes in the technology market place.

The world data standard for these technologies is significant because it will allow smart pack manufacturers to compete with each other on features, rather than on technical standards. This has two major implications:

- The technical interoperability of these devices is assured, so health providers can concentrate on selecting the best device to meet the required patient care objectives.
- The data can be shared between different healthcare record systems, and therefore different health professional groups.

The basic features that will be enabled by Standard 11072–10472 are as follows:

Core Features

- Recording medicine administration events

Optional Features

- Confirming correct usage of medicine
- Subjective patient impressions at the time of administration (how does the patient feel?)
- Storage conditions monitoring
- Anti-tamper mechanism
- Expiry date warning
- Medicine administration reminder

Other areas being considered are interface links with monitoring devices (BP or blood glucose monitoring). At present, there is no plan to include a drug nomenclature in the devices, as development and implementation of an appropriate drug nomenclature standard for these devices would slow down the development and adoption of an overall standard for these devices.

However, while the technologies exist and now a data standard is available, the implications of their implementation have not yet been fully considered by clinicians, health provider organizations and healthcare managers. The business model for adopting these technologies in future will vary around the world, depending on the locality and the healthcare system. It may be that, in some countries, smart packs will be used at source for packaging by the pharmaceutical industry. However in other countries, the technology might be deployed in the pharmacy, with community pharmacy staff packaging medicines into smart packs, just as they now dispense into dosette boxes and other compliance aids.

For example, Apotheker in Germany have industrialised the compliance packaging process, by packing medicines in such "smart" packs for distribution to local pharmacies. A similar model is used by health provider Kaiser Permanente in the United States.

The chief barrier to adoption of these devices is cost. At the time of writing, intelligent blister packs generally cost $7.50 per unit for prototype use, and less than $1 per unit in production. Cost savings are possible for bulk production of these devices, but the cost per unit is still a major limiting factor given the potentially high volume of use of these devices in any health economy. As well as the unit costs of production described above, there are costs associated with the implementation of back-end systems and change in workflow processes. There are also costs associated with the regulatory burden of using these devices. This is certainly an issue where device adoption happens at source in the pharmaceutical industry, as regulatory approval will be needed for each new pack. However, there are likely to be some regulatory and professional issues if these devices are introduced further down the supply chain at the individual pharmacy operator level.

The configuration of the software itself, however, should not be a barrier to deployment of this technology. With the data standard, it will be possible to pre-program the smart pack based on the medicine packaged in it, or alternatively pharmacies could program the smart pack locally according to specific monitoring requirements or agreements with health commissioners.

Specific areas that will need special consideration should these technologies become more widespread are the issue of child safety with the use of these packs and also the question of accessibility by patients with arthritis in their hands or similar disabilities.

Given their potential to revolutionise current pharmacy practice, it is vital that pharmacists are aware of these technologies and are involved with commissioning and piloting of services that utilize them. The health service and commercial pharmacy operators in both the primary care and secondary care sectors will undoubtedly be looking at how these devices could be used to improve the quality of patient care at the institutional level, and device manufacturers will be working with them to pilot these technologies.

However, ultimately these technologies will have an impact on the working lives of pharmacists, and it is vital that pharmacists consider the potential implications.

Pharmacists have a key role in medicine adherence – they see patients more often than doctors about medication-related issues, and the use of "smart" packs would provide pharmacists with more data than has been available previously, on which to base their decisions and advice to patients. Pharmacies are the ideal places for patient compliance to be assessed, as pharmacists are able to see the patient at the point of medicine supply. Pharmacists are primarily involved in the issue of medicines waste, and will be the person most likely to see the medicines that a patient has not taken, when they are returned to the pharmacy, and thus will alerted to a potential compliance issue. Also, pharmacies are a place where monitoring technologies can be supplied (e.g. blood pressure and blood glucose monitoring devices), and these have a place in measuring and supporting adherence and concordance with treatment.

However, there are issues associated with smart pack technology that will determine how these technologies will be used at the point of patient care, and are issues that pharmacists will be closely involved with. The first is the ethical issue concerning consent for the use of the technology. Since the device obtains data from the patient, as they use their medicines, and makes it potentially available to a third party, then from an ethical perspective, the patient will need to give their consent for the smart pack to be used and the data to be gathered, but maybe also specific consent for the data to be made available to a particular healthcare professional. Depending on the healthcare economy, payers may insist on consent being obtained in a particular way.

Another issue is that of acceptability and usability. Patients will prefer using a pack that does not look like a medication pack and that will enable medicines use data to be collected in a way that is as least interruptive as possible to the patient's usual routine. For this reason, the precise physical design of these adherence monitoring packs will be critical to their widespread adoption.

As mentioned, the implementation of smart packs and other adherence monitoring technologies would mean that pharmacists would have access to more data than ever before on patient's medicine-taking behaviours. Apart from the ethical issue about consent, discussed above, pharmacists will be in a position to address medicine-taking behavioural issues in a way that they have not been able to previously. Preliminary evidence of this potential change in practice has been shown in a study of the MEMS device in patients with diabetes [8]. This study showed that feedback from the MEMS device gave more information on medicine-taking behaviour, when compared to manual pill-counting adherence monitoring, and enabled more patient education interventions, before resorting to pharmacological interventions. Pharmacists will therefore need good patient communication skills and may need to develop a different approach to communication about medicine-taking behaviour, which may be based on a coaching and mentoring approach.

Smart packaging will provide data on individual medicine-taking behaviour, and so they will have a major impact on the personalisation of healthcare and the local practice of pharmacists and other healthcare professionals. Since these technologies are centred on the use of medicines, it is essential that the pharmacy profession takes the lead on their implementation. It is to be hoped that pharmacists will be able to debate the issues concerning these technologies and form a consensus about their use before they are introduced by major healthcare providers.

Telecare and Pharmacy

Most of the technology described in the previous section is concerned with streamlining the patient care processes in hospital, and enhancing professional practice. However, an important aspect of modern healthcare is the centrality of the patient in their treatment. As mentioned in earlier chapters, there has been a paradigm shift in the philosophy of healthcare in recent decades, which has been characterised by a number of factors:

(a) the consumerisation of medicine, where governments and health agencies are actively encouraging patients to exercise choice in their medical care, including the choices of therapy and practitioners.
(b) the diminishing paternalism of the medical profession, together with the rise in the autonomy and importance of other health professionals in service delivery, most notably nurses.
(c) the rise in personalized medicine where the use of IT to automate processes can provide medical care that is customized to the individual patient, thus optimizing the quality of care.

There have been many publications describing the role of the "empowered patient" in Twenty-first century healthcare. In England, the Connecting for Health programme sought to embody the principle of patient choice – for example, in the "Choose and Book" appointment booking system. This is likely to continue in future, with the concept of "No choice about me, without me" underpinning NHS reform since 2010 [9], and the recent proposals to improve patient access to electronic medical records [10].

It is clear that a significant area where patients can and should have a greater degree of autonomy, and play an active part in their own care is in the management of chronic diseases. As discussed previously, it is recognised on both sides of the Atlantic that chronic diseases – such as diabetes, asthma and hypertension – are a major cause of increased patient morbidity and reduced quality of life, and therefore are a significant economic burden to the healthcare system. Such diseases are often treated with drugs whose role and pharmacological properties are well-established, but which require regular monitoring, and the most significant factor in the cost of these diseases is the cost of hospitalisation and acute treatment for a patient whose disease has become uncontrolled.

American commentators have identified the huge potential of EP systems to contribute to evidence-based medicine in patients with chronic diseases [11]. However, at the current time, in the US, EP systems are used in a small proportion of acute hospitals. There is therefore very little experience, if any at all, in the use of secondary care EP systems to gather monitoring data for patients with chronic diseases, either from GP systems (primary care systems) or from remote devices. This is a potentially major area of expansion for secondary care EP systems. There is the possibility that a healthcare provider based EP system might become the "hub" for care of chronic diseases in a series of patient populations in the community – for example, diabetes, asthma or hypertension – across a region, as shown in Fig. 8.2.

Appropriate technology – such as the internet, digital televisions and mobile phones would be used to support and enable the patient, as they take responsibility for their day-to-day self-care at home and in the community. Healthcare IT researchers have identified the potential of the electronic health record as a means of empowering the patient and supporting care process involvement [12, 13].

Fig. 8.2 Pharmacy IT as a
"hub" for chronic disease
management

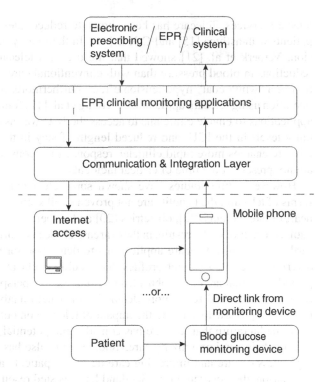

Examples of telecare technology would include the following:

- Use of a mobile phone to submit blood glucose readings to a diabetes care module of an EP system. Warnings concerning the amendment of the monitoring schedule or the insulin regimen would then be automatically calculated and sent back to the patient via SMS text message.
- Use of a digital television in the patient's home to allow the patient to log on to patient monitoring web facilities to view graphical monitoring information on their disease.

While telecare to enable patients to manage chronic diseases might, at first sight, appear to be a form of device integration, telecare involves a wider range of device modalities and manufacturers than might be found in the acute clinical environment. Consequently, research in this area involves the coordination of a variety of stakeholders and is much more in its infancy, compared to system integration within the acute sector.

The remainder of this section will review literature which has evaluated telecare applications for the management of chronic diseases. Telecare services of different types have now been established in a range of therapeutic areas, including stroke [14], respiratory diseases [15, 16] remote intensive care unit (ICU) operation [17], palliative care [18, 19] obstetrics [20] and cardiovascular diseases [21, 22]. In some of these areas, evaluations have shown clear outcome benefits with the use of certain telecare services. Telecare has been shown to reduce rates of hospital admission in patients with asthma [15] and COPD [16]. In their study of patients with hypertension, Verberk et al. [21] showed that the use of a telecare service led to greater reductions in blood pressure than with conventional care, possibly due to a reduction in a "white coat" hypertension effect. Furthermore, in a study of remote ICU operation using telecare applications, Young et al. [17] found that the use of telecare applications to enable clinicians to access the ICU was associated with lower mortality levels in the ICU, and reduced length of stay in the ICU, probably because telecare enables more rapid clinician response than conventional care, if clinicians are not present at the time of critical incidents.

However, while studies have shown some clear outcome benefits with some forms of telecare, the benefits are not proven in all scenarios. Reviews of telecare in heart failure patients [22], obstetrics [20] and diabetes [23] have commented on the equivocal nature of the results in these areas. These and various other studies call for further research in telecare applications to determine further outcome benefits, to determine the exact patient profiles that would benefit from these services, and to provide data that are more robust from a study design perspective. In addition, some reviews have called for a more detailed cost-benefit analysis of telecare services, [15, 24–26]. Notwithstanding the impact of telecare on outcome benefits, it is clear from the literature that telecare has considerable potential for improving personalized medicine and optimizing care. Telemedicine also has the potential for extending access to care and improving care access to patients in isolated locations. For this reason, the government of Scotland has invested resources into evaluating telecare for provision of enhanced healthcare services to residents of the Highlands and islands of Scotland. As well as access to healthcare for patients, reductions in traveling times for patients, staff and visitors are clear social and economic benefits of telecare. The Scottish Government established a telecare development programme, with the following objectives:

1. Reduction of the number of avoidable emergency admissions and readmissions to hospital;
2. Increase in the speed of discharge from hospital once clinical need is met;
3. Reduction of the use of care homes;
4. Improvement of the quality of life of users of telecare services;
5. Reduction of the pressure on (informal) carers;
6. Extension of the range of people assisted by telecare services in Scotland;
7. Realisation of efficiencies (cash releasing or time releasing) from the investment in telecare;
8. Support for effective procurement to ensure that telecare services grow as quickly as possible.

A final report of the programme was published in 2009 [27] and provides detailed information on how the objectives have been met, and where further progress is needed.

Telemedicine is beneficial in patients with poor mobility, such as spinal cord injuries and disorders [28], elderly and housebound patients [29] or those for whom the optimum care setting is their own home, such as palliative care patients [18]. Telecare modalities will also provide the basis for services that enable more patients to be treated without attending hospital – for example, outpatient parenteral antibiotics [30].

A number of studies have been conducted with the use of telemedicine software on mobile phones to help patients with the management and monitoring of chronic diseases [31], such as asthma and diabetes (Anhoj et al. [32], Farmer et al. [33]). These applications provided the advantage of real time uploading of monitoring information, and therefore in theory, a more accurate record of patient response to therapy. However, in these studies, the display of monitoring data on the phone screen was difficult to read for patients.

Gammon et al. [34] studied the use of a system which transferred the blood glucose results for a child, from the child's blood glucose testing device to a parent's mobile phone. The aim of the study was to conduct a preliminary assessment of the feasibility and use of the system, and the study was conducted with a group of 15 young people, between 9 and 15 years of age. The system was found to be easy to use, but its value was primarily as a means of reassurance for the parents; issues arose with the system concerning the independence and autonomy of the young person, and their attitude to parental control. Young people who were good at monitoring their blood glucose levels found that, with the system, the number of parental reminders was reduced, because the parents had evidence of the child's compliance with the monitoring requirement. As might be expected, for children who were less reliable at monitoring their blood glucose, the use of the system increased the number of parental interventions. The authors commented, however, that increased parental monitoring did not necessarily lead to improved glycaemic control, since it often led to conflict between the parent and the child, which had a negative effect on monitoring compliance.

Telecare has the potential to provide considerable benefits to well-motivated patients who are committed to monitoring their chronic diseases, and to the healthcare professionals that support them. In particular, real-time monitoring information feeds from stand-alone testing devices, or domiciliary telemedicine monitoring systems have the potential to contribute to decision support functions in EP systems both in the hospital and in the community. The interface of such systems with hospital EP systems, so that hospital clinicians can obtain a clear and reliable record of recent monitoring results (e.g. blood glucose readings with diabetes), may enable patients to be treated more efficiently in hospital for complications or relapses of their chronic diseases.

There are a number of barriers to adoption of telemedicine systems. They are as follows:

1. Lack of a generic dataset. A feature of many telemedicine prototypes is that their datasets are proprietary, and are specific to a particular device manufacturer. Work has recently been conducted on the development of a generic dataset, based on XML messaging, which can be used for a variety of devices and applications [35].

2. The willingness of stakeholders to cooperate in system development. The development of such systems, together with their prototyping and testing, will require close collaboration between a wide range of stakeholders, including clinical professionals, health informatics specialists, Hospital IM&T professionals, together with software and hardware/device vendors.
3. The availability of funding for telecare services and the availability of appropriate evidence to support business cases to secure funding. These issues are being addressed by the current literature available but, as discussed, further work is needed on the cost-effectiveness issues.
4. The adoption of such modalities by patients and clinical professionals. As discussed in Chap. 1, it is recognised that there is an adoption curve to a change or innovation. Depending on personality and worldviews, some individuals will embrace a change of procedure willingly, whereas others will be reluctant. Indeed, the greater the potential impact on a new technology on a patient's personal life – and a near-patient telemedicine monitoring system can have a potentially major impact on a patient's way of life – the more information and reassurance a patient will need to adopt a new technology or procedure. Patient attitudes to disease and illness will also be a factor. Some patients will not want to be "empowered" in the treatment of their illness; they would rather be passive and leave responsibility for treatment with a healthcare professional.
5. Ethical issues associated with these technologies. The ethical issues with "smart" packaging would also, to some extent, apply to telecare; patients would need to give explicit consent for data to be collected, if it was not obvious that this was happening, and some patients might not want their data to be shared with other healthcare professionals. Telecare also raises ethical questions concerning the cost-effectiveness of service provision with expensive telecare modalities, the disengagement of patients from healthcare professionals as a result of telemedicine and how this affects clinical practice, and the suitability of systems for different patient groups (for example, children and the elderly)

Clinical Homecare

Related to telecare, where clinical consultation, diagnosis and disease monitoring may be provided directly to the patient's home via video and telecommunications technology, is clinical homecare, where a treatment is provided to the patient in their own home (either self-administered or administered by a health professional as part of the service). Clinical homecare is now widespread in the UK and US, and provides significant benefits in provision of therapy without the costs of outpatient or day case hospital attendance, and delivery of care in a way that is convenient and more acceptable to patients. However, it is a complex discipline requiring input from several stakeholders, typically an acute healthcare provider, a pharmaceutical company and the homecare company that actually delivers the therapy service. For this reason, the regulatory requirements are complicated – a homecare provider company may be simultaneously a registered pharmacy, a pharmaceutical manufacturer and a nursing care provider, and would need to comply with the relevant regulations [36]. Because of multiple stakeholders in homecare services and the use of different homecare companies for different services even by the same healthcare provider organization, a recent England Department of Health (DH) review has highlighted issues concerning the transparency of commissioning processes, a need for more robust governance by clinical leads in provider organizations and more regional coordination [37].

EP systems have the potential to support commissioning and governance of homecare services, if there are appropriate interfaces with homecare company IT systems and information systems to support commissioning. The England DH review has indicated that links with EP systems and standard pharmacy management systems are required to optimize homecare services [38].

Methodology and Evaluation

Quantitative studies on electronic prescribing and other medicines management IT systems are designed to perform a statistical analysis on error rates and other risk issues in the medicines management process, and to evaluate the system as an intervention in the process. However, there are various confounding factors with quantitative evaluations, which may include the following:

(a) the subjectivity of reviewers in the evaluation of adverse drug events and medication errors in these studies;
(b) the lack of parallel studies between units with EP and those without EP in the same hospital;
(c) the extent to which the study period represents the full implementation schedule of the EP system. If certain functions of an EP system are not available, this may have a profound effect on the error rates detected by a quantitative study.
(d) error detection bias in error reporting, due to the vigilance of researchers and users when evaluating a new system, and
(e) the extent to which the benefits reported are specific to the working practices of the sites studied.

The extent to which these confounding factors associated with research methodology or system design affect benefits needs to be evaluated in more detail.

A number of papers have commented on the methodology of quantitative evaluations of EP systems. In a systematic review, Ammenwerth et al. [39] noted that, while EP systems can reduce the risk of medication errors, quantitative studies varied considerably in their setting, design, quality and results. The authors called for more randomized controlled trial methodology covering a wider range of clinical settings and geographical locations. Similarly, following their review of EP studies, Reckmann et al. [40] called for greater control of EP study conditions, larger sample sizes and standardized definitions of error types.

It has been suggested [41] that there should be a formal methodology for validation of EP software, analogous to the process of licensing a new medicine. However, while a prospective, controlled study is the "gold standard" in clinical medicine, and especially therapeutics, to demonstrate associations and causal links, such studies are much harder to design to assess clinical informatics interventions.

In his discussion of the methodologies for evaluation of EP systems, Trent Rosenbloom [42] describes a number of problems in the design of clinical informatics studies, including (a) the isolations of specific system variables to be tested, (b) the choice of the most appropriate units of study (individual patient, ward, consultant list or hospital) to be exposed to the system variable under study conditions, and (c) ensuring that the study groups remain distinct during the time that systems or workflows are tested, and that there is no inadvertent cross-over of subjects.

While there is a clear need for quantitative data on the operation of EP systems, the insights that qualitative techniques can provide should not be discounted. Savage et al. [43] compared medication error rate pictures obtained by quantitative and qualitative methods at an English hospital after implementation of an EP system. They concluded that, while the two processes provided an similar picture of the drug use process, interviews took less time to conduct than retrospective record review (and were therefore more cost-effective), provided more information on the prescribing process, identified two errors that were not found in record review and provided reasons for delayed or omitted administration of medicines.

Development of Professional Standards

As discussed in Chap. 1, a variety of coding systems have been developed to enable information about medicines to be transmitted in a machine-readable manner, and these coding systems are the building blocks of technology use for medicines management applications, and also technical and functional integration between different systems.

However, in pharmacy and prescribing, there is a need for professional standards for electronic systems which set requirements for standard datasets and system functions to support the professional best practice needed to ensure optimum patient safety, high quality of care and efficient use of resources. If professional bodies do not lead on the development of professional standards for systems, there is the risk that the availability and usabilty of pharmacy IT functionality will be determined by the development plans of software vendors, and driven by their commercial priorities, rather than the needs of the service and of patient care.

However, it is simplistic to say that this is an either/or situation. As with other businesses, software vendors formulate their development plans at least partly in response to their customer needs, to ensure revenue streams from ongoing sales and upgrades. Consequently, if pharmacy users need changes in functionality to support best practice, then in the ideal world, these requirements would find their way onto the development roadmap for system vendors. However, as discussed previously, the business model of pharmacy system development in UK community pharmacy (i.e. as a subsidised offering from a wholesaler) has not been conducive for a healthy customer relationship, where pharmacy users drive the adoption of the most appropriate functionality.

Nevertheless, if the development of functional requirements is left purely to commercial pressures, there is the danger that proprietary features will develop to enable software vendors to leverage the competition, and this will lead to inconsistency in functionality between systems and reduced potential for intraoperability between systems.

The best approach is where professional bodies engage with suppliers, and suppliers engage with professional bodies, to ensure the development of effective and achievable standards. Professional bodies will necessarily lead the development of professional standards, but the input of suppliers is vital, as suppliers have the necessary knowledge of technical and infrastucture limitations necessary for developing the required functionality, and will have to deliver it in a way that is consistent with their commercial needs.

In the UK, the Royal College of Physicians has led a number of workstreams to develop professional standards for medical record keeping, for example, its work on standard format and content for hospital admission and discharge records [44], and work on core clinical headings on medical records. As previously discussed, good management of the discharge process is important for hospitals and appropriate communication of information is necessary to ensure continuity of care when the patient is transferred from one care setting to another. The Royal Pharmaceutical Society's Transfer of Care guidance [45] includes a core dataset for information on medication which should be communicated from one healthcare provider to another.

As previously discussed, there is a need for a standard for the record format and content that meets requirements for pharmaceutical care. Some of the required data items will be the same as in record requirements for medicine, for example the Royal College of Physicians record standards, and any standards developed for pharmacy would need to be consistent with the requirements for other professions. However, there are some concepts about medicines, for example relating to delivery devices, compliance aids and specific administration instructions, that will be specific to pharmacy practice, and would not be of interest to other professional groups. There is a need to ensure that all of these concepts can be described in a machine-readable way, and in a record format which supports patient centred pharmaceutical care by the pharmacy team according to accepted best practice.

Considerable research has been done on pharmaceutical care records in the US [46]. However, no professional standards have emerged as yet in the UK, although over the last few years, the Royal Pharmaceutical Society has been conducting work to establish a framework for a standard pharmaceutical care record. At the time of writing, this work is ongoing.

For professional standards to be developed in pharmacy, there is an essential process of meaningful engagement with the various sectors of the pharmacy profession, to ensure that standards meet their specific needs and that they therefore have ownership of the emerging standards. However, in the UK and many other countries, the pharmacy profession is highly fragmented, in terms of the number of pharmacy bodies and associations, and there are a range of views concerning the adoption of technology in general, and its use in healthcare in particular. These issues mean that a great deal of work needs to be done to persuade pharmacists of the benefits and utility of IT in pharmacy practice, and of how risks can be mitigated, before any IT implementation and change management can take place.

Pharmacy Professional Engagement in IT Adoption

A vital aspect of the development of IT to support pharmacy practice is the engagement of the pharmacy profession (professional engagement) with the adoption and use of technologies to support current roles and enable new roles. At present, only a small proportion of the pharmacy profession is engaged with, and supportive of, the use of IT systems for routine pharmacy practice and development of new roles. While this is consistent with the adoption of innovations in any sphere of activity [47], this inertia with professional engagement does raise particular problems. Often healthcare IT engagement events are attended by a small number of IT enthusiasts from the profession, rather than the broad consensus of professionals which would be needed to secure adoption of a technology within the profession. Often, those with the time and availability to attend IT engagement events are not representative of their profession and may give IT implementers an unrealistic view of professional issues. However, a much larger proportion of the pharmacy profession – including those who are professional leaders and clinical opinion formers – would need to adopt IT use in routine practice for widespread IT use to become part of the professional culture.

In addition, there are issues surrounding the extent to which technological change is driven by systems or people. It is tempting to assume that information technology will effortlessly provide the infrastructure and functions to support the new roles for pharmacists, and that all that is required to adopt these roles is install and use software and systems that will support them. However, this systems-based approach will lead to a flawed service, which will provide poor patient care and will be rightly rejected by the pharmacy profession. This is for two reasons. Firstly, reliance on an IT system for service provision raises the risk that the service will be retro-engineered to fit the functions and capability of the software, rather than be structured to meet the needs of the patient. Secondly, if a pharmacist uses an IT system to facilitate or support a pharmacy service, there is a danger that the onus of responsibility for the service will be insidiously shifted onto the system, when the pharmacist ultimately remains professionally accountable for it. This will lead to a diminishing of the pharmacist's role, disempowerment of the pharmacist in the healthcare system and, of course, decreased job satisfaction. This second issue is important and deserves further exploration in a wider context.

In a controversial paper published in 2007 [48] US economist Michael Porter described how, in order to develop the best value health service, service development must be clinician-led. He argued that Government health reforms typically were imposed on clinicians from outside their professions, had as their only goal healthcare cost reduction, and were incremental in their nature. Such approaches created a "zero sum" health system where resources allocated to one patient were often made available at the expense of another patient, leading to increased stress and reduced job satisfaction for the health professionals concerned.

Porter argued that any health strategy should be clinician-led, and based on three principles: (a) the goal of healthcare should be good value for patients, not cost reduction; (b) healthcare practice should be organized around patient health needs and care cycles and – crucially – (c) results and outcomes must be rigorously measured in order to influence future service development. This approach leads to a "positive sum" health system, where the value to the patient is the ultimate outcome measure, where there is healthy competition and where beneficial innovation is rewarded.

While these observations are based on the US healthcare system, there are some striking parallels with the situation facing UK pharmacists, who are moving towards provision of patient-focused services, based on specific medical conditions and cycles of care, rather than a service based purely on the supply of medicines. There is a clear argument, then, that pharmacists as health professionals will need to lead the pharmacy services that they develop. Pharmacists will need to take responsibility for formulating the business models for these services and, as necessary, leveraging the funding from commissioners. And – most significantly – pharmacists will need to actively decide what IT systems and functions they will need to support the best value healthcare services for their patients, rather than allow these functions to be defined for them by software vendors.

Service development begins with the commitment of health professionals to their patients, which is essentially an interpersonal relationship and, while technology undoubtedly has a place in service provision, no software package or IT system alone can replace wise and patient focused professional leadership.

There are good reasons why any health profession should engage with the use of IT to support their professional activities. If systems implemented do not support professional activities, then the following situations can arise:

1. Inefficiencies in recording service user information if terms used by the profession cannot be quickly and accurately selected
2. Failure to code patient information so that it can also be used in the national research databases to facilitate multi-site and local research studies and greatly increase the pace of accumulation of evidence of effectiveness of care.
3. Having to use electronic care pathways designed without pharmacy input.
4. Having to use generic Care Planning modules

There are many reasons for the inertia associated with professional engagement with IT adoption and use. Some of the reasons for the pharmacy profession are as follows:

1. Senior pharmacists are not engaged with the use of technology for service development or, if they are, they are not senior enough in health provider organizations to facilitate actual implementation of change.
2. Managers of pharmacists within health provider organizations and pharmacy businesses do not support them in professional engagement activities.
3. Senior pharmacists cannot spend time in service strategy planning due to inability to get locum cover, or because of other service priorities.
4. Pharmacy professional bodies may not hear about, or recognise the importance of, technology change and healthcare IT development strategies.
5. Pharmacists may focus on the pressures of their day-to-day workload and find it hard to prioritise engagement activities that require a reflective and developmental approach
6. Pharmacists may not regard the development of new IT systems as a local service priority.

Nevertheless, professional engagement with pharmacy IT as a means of supporting current practice and developing new practice is essential if the pharmacy profession is to develop to meet its aspirations and to ensure that its value is recognized by patients, other healthcare professionals and policy makers.

IT Education and Training

The importance of training and orientation in healthcare IT for healthcare professionals has emerged gradually over the last decade, and while much has been achieved in this area, there is more to be done. Training on specific IT systems is quite rightly the responsibility of systems vendors, as they will need to ensure that their user training addresses system-specific functionality and takes into account system-specific enhancements and developments. However, because of the way that IT has developed over the last 30 years, during the working life of many current pharmacy professionals, there is a real need for education and orientation on basic IT skills, in a way that is appropriate to the professional group.

Training and education in healthcare IT for pharmacists is important for the following reasons:

- It encourages pharmacists to see the benefits and risks of using IT systems, and to evaluate them from a perspective of professional accountability
- It helps to model best practice in the profession, and encourages a culture of ownership of IT systems in the practice environment
- It can be used to deliver other aspects of pharmacy education and professional development.
- It can provide pharmacists with a range of basic IT skills, gained in the professional environment but which may transferrable to other areas of life.

The report *Learning to Manage Health Information* was first published in 1999 [49] and established a common health informatics framework for healthcare professionals at pre and post-registration level. It included learning outcomes and standards for professional practice under eight themes covering areas of learning in health informatics, including protection of individuals and organizations, data, information and knowledge, coding and terminology, care records and clinical systems and applications

This framework concentrated on the essential learning outcomes that need to be incorporated into educational programmes, and gave guidance on the level of clinical education at which outcomes should be embedded (e.g. basic qualification, post first qualification/CPD, advanced and specialist practice). The emphasis was that informatics should not be taught as a distinct subject but should be embedded (embedding of clinical informatics) and woven into the whole clinical curriculum. This work led to the establishment of the eICE programme (embedding Informatics in Clinical Education) by NHS Connecting for Health, to encourage the incorporation of informatics training into the clinical education process.

This approach has been accepted by many healthcare professions. Various pharmacy continuing professional development (CPD) providers in the UK have integrated their IT learning into the general curriculum. Consequently, for each therapeutic area or pharmacy service CPD module, providers have included the specific IT issues for that service in the module, rather than delivering pharmacy IT CPD as a separate stream. This approach is beneficial as it helps professionals to follow a reflective CPD cycle and to contextualize their learning in practice.

Nevertheless, the lack of basic IT knowledge and skills in certain parts of the healthcare workforce is a major barrier to IT engagement and adoption. In the UK in recent years, the NHS has developed two initiatives to address this issue. These are the NHS eLearning IT Essentials (NHS ELITE) and the NHS eLearning for Health Information Systems (NHS Health), both accredited by the British Computer Society.

NHS ELITE covers generic IT skills, and NHS Health covers information governance, data protection, and patient confidentiality in the NHS. As with other healthcare professionals, it is essential that all members of the pharmacy team are competent to use technologies in their workplace. This includes not only well-established system like pharmacy systems, but also the technologies that will support new services such as electronic health records, telecare, automation and mobile devices. As well as understanding the hardware and software, users should have an understanding of the relevant governance and legal issues (e.g. consent to share information, and confidentiality of personal information). As well as these initiatives, NHS Connecting for Health has also supported the European Computer Driving License initiative, which provides basic IT skills training to individuals, regardless of professional group and industry sector. These basic IT skills learning initiatives have been criticized by certain parts of the pharmacy profession as being too simplistic and removed from specialist pharmacy practice. However, they may have a major role to play in promoting engagement with IT issues by a diverse range of healthcare staff, and developing the basic IT skills required to operate safely and effectively in the clinical environment.

While efforts are being made to ensure that pharmacy professionals receive appropriate training and orientation about the use of IT in their practice in general, there is still much to be done on the development of a clinical IT training and education strategy across the pharmacy profession, including:

- Undergraduate & Pre-registration training
- Early Career Development
- Continuing Professional Development
- Revalidation/Renewal of Licensure
- IT education to support advanced and specialist practice in clinical disciplines
- Pharmacy Informatics Specialist Pharmacy Training

In 2007, in the US, the Accreditation Council for Pharmacy Education (ACPE) introduced a requirement that entry level Doctor of Pharmacy candidates had to demonstrate expertise in informatics. Also the American Society of Health System Pharmacists (ASHP) have developed learning objectives for a pharmacy informatics residency programme. Consequently, the American Pharmacists' Association (APA) formulated a set of core competencies in pharmacy informatics, which have been published as a textbook [50] for pharmacists as part of their general training. These competencies cover:

- IT basics – fundamentals of computing, networking and telecommunications, data management and communications standards/interoperability.
- Computerised Physician Order Entry (CPOE), electronic prescribing.
- Clinical Decision Support (CDS) systems.
- Pharmacy information systems.
- Electronic health records.
- Pharmacy automation.
- The contextualization of pharmacy IT systems into pharmacy practice.

These competencies aim to explore the use of pharmacy IT in the context of professional practice, not as a technical discipline, although textbook material of a purely technical nature (e.g. communications standards) tends to become outdated quickly. However, these competencies provide a good framework of healthcare IT knowledge for generalist pharmacists training for specialist roles in clinical pharmacy, and there is currently no equivalent competence framework for clinical pharmacy training in the UK.

The other area where further development is required is the establishment of a distinct career progression for pharmacists wishing to specialise in pharmacy informatics. At the current time, many pharmacists who specialise in pharmacy informatics enter the field through specific employment experience as part of a general role (e.g. implementing a hospital electronic prescribing system), and there is no coordinated system of training and qualification in health informatics. In the US, this has been addressed in part by the work done by AHSP section of pharmacy informatics and technology on pharmacy informatics residencies and provision of coordination and resources on pharmacy informatics.

However, there is no similar career progression for informatics specialist pharmacists in the UK. The UK Chartered Health Informatics Professional (UKCHIP) initiative launched by the eICE programme consists of competences and a basic accreditation framework for health informatics professionals, and thus provides an appropriate specialist training for healthcare professionals involved in informatics. However, it is not specific to pharmacy. Furthermore, the British Computer Society offers courses and specialist memberships in healthcare informatics. It is to be hoped that in future, there would be a more coordinated approach to pharmacy informatics specialisation within the pharmacy profession by stakeholder organisations in the UK and elsewhere in Europe.

Conclusion

Various systems and devices have been developed to manage the medicines use process, including electronic health records, prescribing and medicines management systems, pharmacy management systems, and pharmacy automation. The available literature suggests that, as individual systems, these applications have the potential to provide benefits to pharmacists and their patients, in terms of reduction of medication-related errors, and improvement of workflow efficiencies. However, there is a need for research into integrated systems to ascertain their total benefits on the medicine use process. There is also a need to evaluate new technologies, such as smart infusion pumps and smart packaging, which may have a major impact on current working practices, not to mention ethical implications. In any case, as well as technological adoption and innovation, pharmacists and pharmacy managers have much work to do at a professional and policy level, to encourage engagement in IT adoption, training and education in clinical IT and development of professional standards to ensure that pharmacy IT systems have the greatest impact on patient care.

References

1. Connecting for Health. E-prescribing functional specification for NHS Trusts. 2007. http:/www.connectingforhealth.nhs.uk/systemsandservices/eprescribing. p. 125–6. Accessed on Apr 2012.
2. Hunt DL, Haynes RB, et al. Effects of computer-based clinical decision support systems on physician performance and patient outcomes: a systematic review. JAMA. 1998;280:1339–46.
3. Husch M, Sullivan C, et al. Insights from the sharp end of intravenous medication errors: implications for infusion pump technology. Qual Saf Health Care. 2005;14:80–6.
4. Kripalani S, Yao X, Haynes RB. Interventions to enhance medication adherence in chronic medical conditions: a systematic review. Arch Intern Med. 2007;167(6):540–50.
5. Garfield S, Barber N, Walley P, Willson A, Eliasson L. Quality of medication use in primary care – mapping the problem, working to a solution: a systematic review of the literature. BMC Med. 2009;7:50.
6. Saini SD, Schoenfeld P, Kaulback K, Dubinsky MC. Effect of medication dosing frequency on adherence in chronic diseases. Am J Manag Care. 2009;15(6):22–33.
7. Goundrey-Smith SJ. Principles of electronic prescribing. London: Springer; 2008. p. 142.
8. Matsuyama JR, Mason BJ, Jue SG. Pharmacists' interventions using an electronic medication monitoring device's adherence data versus pill counts. Ann Pharmacother. 1993;27(7–8):851–5.

9. England Department of Health. Equity and excellence: liberating the NHS. 2010. p. 3 http://www.dh.gov.uk/en/Publicationsandstatistics/Publications/PublicationsPolicyAndGuidance/DH_117353. Accessed on Apr 2012.
10. England Department of Health. An information revolution. 2010. p. 18. http://www.dh.gov.uk/prod_consum_dh/groups/dh_digitalassets/@dh/@en/documents/digitalasset/dh_120598.pdf. Accessed on Apr 2012.
11. Shane R. Computerised physician order entry: challenges and opportunities. Am J Health Syst Pharm. 2002;59:286–8.
12. Knaup P, Bott O, et al. Electronic Patient Records: moving from islands and bridges towards Electronic Health Records for continuity of care. Methods Inf Med. 2007;46 Suppl 1:34–46.
13. Ueckert F, Goerz M, et al. Empowerment of patients and communication with healthcare professionals through an electronic health record. Int J Med Inform. 2003;70:99–108.
14. Stewart SF, Switzer JA. Perspectives on telemedicine to improve stroke treatment. Drugs Today (Barc). 2011;47:157–67.
15. McLean S, Chandler D, et al. Telehealthcare for asthma: a Cochrane review. Can Med Assoc J. 2011;183:E733–42.
16. McLean S, Nurmatov U, et al. Telehealthcare for chronic obstructive pulmonary disease. Cochrane Database Syst Rev. 2011;(7):CD007718.
17. Young LB, Chan PS, et al. Impact of telemedicine intensive care unit coverage on patient outcomes: a systematic review and metaanalysis. Arch Intern Med. 2011;171:498–506.
18. Johnston B. UK telehealth initiatives in palliative care: a review. Int J Palliat Nurs. 2011;17:301–8.
19. Kidd L, Cayless S, et al. Telehealth in palliative care in the UK: a review of the evidence. J Telemed Telecare. 2010;16:394–402.
20. Magann EF, McKelvey SS, et al. The use of telemedicine in obstetrics: a review of the literature. Obstet Gynecol Surv. 2011;66:170–8.
21. Verberk WJ, Kessels AG, et al. Telecare is a valuable tool for hypertension management, a systematic review and meta-analysis. Blood Press Monit. 2011;16:149–55.
22. Anker SD, Koehler F, et al. Telemedicine and remote management of patients with heart failure. Lancet. 2011;378:731–9.
23. Costa BM, Fitzgerald KJ, et al. Effectiveness of IT-based diabetes management interventions: a review of the literature. BMC Fam Pract. 2009;10:72.
24. Ekeland AG, Bowes A, et al. Effectiveness of telemedicine: a systematic review of reviews. Int J Med Inform. 2010;79:736–71.
25. Gaikwad R, Warren J. The role of home-based information and communications technology interventions in chronic disease management: a systematic literature review. Health Informatics J. 2009;15:122–46.
26. Vitacca M, Mazzu M, et al. Sociotechnical and organisational challenges to wider e-health implementation. Chron Respir Dis. 2009;6:91–7.
27. Scottish Telemedicine Report. http://www.jitscotland.org.uk/action-areas/telecare-in-scotland/.
28. Woo C, Guihan M, et al. What's happening now! Telehealth management of spinal cord injuries/disorders. J Spinal Cord Med. 2011;34(3):322–31.
29. Koch S, Hagglund M. Health informatics and the delivery of care to older people. Maturitas. 2009;63:195–9.
30. Eron L. Telemedicine: the future of outpatient therapy. Clin Infect Dis. 2010;51 Suppl 2:S224–30.
31. Mc William S. How mobiles and pharmacy are set to revolutionise chronic disease treatment. Pharm J. 2006;276:7–8.
32. Anhoj J, Moldrup C. Feasability of collecting diary data from asthma patient mobile phones and SMS (short message service): review analysis and focus group evaluation from a pilot study. J Med Internet Res. 2004;6:e42.
33. Farmer AJ, Gibson OJ, et al. A randomised controlled trial of the effect of real-time telemedicine support on glycaemic control in young adults with type 1 diabetes. Diabetes Care. 2005;28:2697–702.

34. Gammon D, Arsand E, et al. Parent–child interaction using a mobile and wireless system for blood glucose monitoring. J Med Internet Res. 2005;5:e57.
35. Di Giacomo P, Ricci FL. Generic data modelling and use of XML standard for home telemonitoring of chronically ill patients. Stud Health Technol Inform. 2002;90:163–7.
36. Payne N. Presented at the National Clinical Homecare Association Conference, Birmingham, Oct 2011. http://www.clinicalhomecare.co.uk/images/stories/documents/presentations/nick_payne.pdf. Accessed on Apr 2012.
37. Hackett M. Homecare medicines: towards a vision for the future. England Department of Health; 2010. p. 6–18. http://cmu.dh.gov.uk/homecare-medicines-review-group. Accessed on Apr 2012.
38. Hackett M. Homecare medicines: towards a vision for the future. England Department of Health; 2010. p. 10–51. http://cmu.dh.gov.uk/homecare-medicines-review-group. Accessed on Apr 2012.
39. Ammenwerth E, Schnell-Inderst P, et al. The effect of electronic prescribing on medication errors and adverse drug events: a systematic review. J Am Med Inform Assoc. 2008;15:585–600.
40. Reckmann MH, Westbrook JI, Koh Y, Lo C, Day RO. Does computerised provider order entry reduce prescribing errors for hospital inpatients? A systematic review. J Am Med Inform Assoc. 2009;16:613–23.
41. Summers V. Association of Scottish Chief Pharmacists. Electronic prescribing – the way forward. Pharm J. 2000;265:834.
42. Trent Rosenbloom S. Approaches to evaluating electronic prescribing. J Am Med Inform Assoc. 2006;13:399–401.
43. Savage I, Cornford T, Klecun E, Barber N, Clifford S, Franklin BD. Medication errors with electronic prescribing (EP): two views of the same picture. BMC Health Serv Res. 2010;10:135.
44. Royal College of Physicians. Developing standards for the structure and content of health records. London. 2008. www.rcplondon.ac.uk/clinical-standards/hiu/medical-records.
45. Royal Pharmaceutical Society. Keeping patients safe when they transfer between care providers – getting the medicines right: Good practice guidance for healthcare professions. 2011. http://www.rpharms.com/medicines-safety/getting-the-medicines-right.asp. Accessed on Sep 2012.
46. Hepler CD, Strand LM. Opportunities and Responsibilities in Pharmaceutical Care. Am J Hosp Pharm. 1990;47(3):533–43.
47. Rogers EM. Diffusions of Innvoation. 5th Ed. 2005. New York. Free Press, p22.
48. Porter ME, Teisberg EO. How physicians can change the future of healthcare. JAMA. 2007;297(10):1103–11.
49. LtMHI. http://www.connectingforhealth.nhs.uk/systemsandservices/capability/health/hidcurriculum/brochure.pdf. Accessed on Apr 2012.
50. Fox BI, Thrower MR, et al. Building core competencies in pharmacy informatics. Washington, D.C.: American Pharmacists Association; 2010.

Appendices

Appendix A: Glossary of Terms

Barcode a form of data carrier where data are represented by a symbology which may be scanned optically.

Biometric ID system which confirms a person's identification by biometric means – for example, by finger-print or retinal scan.

Data carrier a way of representing data in a machine readable form. A barcode is a data carrier

Data Standard a convention for the structure and format of types of data

Data migration the process of transferring the data from an existing system to a new and different system

dm + d the NHS Connecting for Health terminology service for medicines

EAN (European Article Number) Code open, global data standards for product, patient, location and asset ID.

Electronic Data Interchange (EDI) the ability to enter and transmit information in electronic form, either by direct connection or via a modem.

Electronic health record (EHR) an electronic record of the patient's entire healthcare history (including prescribing history).

ePharmacy the service for electronic transfer of prescriptions and IT support for other pharmacy services in Scotland

Electronic Prescribing (EP) systems systems for prescribing medicines electronically in hospitals (may be referred to as computerised physician order entry (CPOE) in US)

Electronic Prescription Service (EPS) the NHS Connecting for Health service for electronic transfer of prescriptions (eTP) in the community in England.

Electronic Transfer of Prescriptions (eTP) the use of computer systems to generate, transmit and receive electronic prescriptions in primary care

Electronic point of sale (EPOS) system electronic system used to support sales transactions and merchandising in a retail environment (electronic cash registers)

Global Trade Item Number (GTIN) a numerical identifier to enable transport or storage of products at different points in the supply chain. This is the EAN Code

Intraoperability the process ensuring that pharmacy IT systems can communicate with each other in an effective way.

Metadata the data that are ancillary to a patient record – for example, an audit log of dates and times when the record was amended, and by whom.

PIP code a human readable coding method for pharmacy products. Used in the transmission of order information between pharmacy and wholesaler (and others).

Primary Care Trusts current payor bodies for primary care health services in the UK National Health Service. Following the NHS reforms, they will be abolished and many of their roles will be taken on by Clinical Commissioning Groups.

Radio Frequency Identification (RFID) a means of product and asset identification and tracking using a microchip tag queried by a radio frequency reader

Smart card personal permission card for accessing patient data on the NHS Connecting for Health spine.

SNOMED Clinical Terms (SNOMED CT) universal healthcare devices and medicines terminology. http://www.snomed.org/

Standard Pharmaceutical Care Record (SPhCR) a proposed standard dataset to enable pharmaceutical care, which would be incorporated in EHRs.

Summary Care Record the NHS Connecting for Health EHR system in England

Symbology a convention for representing numeric or alphabetic data in an optical form

Telehealth or telecare the use of interactive video technology to enable remote provision of care

Appendix B: Data Fields for Pharmaceutical Care

Patient Demographic Data
(*Basic dataset*)

Patient Details
- Age
- Weight
- Gender

GP Details
- GP details
- Recent visit(s) to GP
- Any recent referrals (including GP, AE, MIU visits), to whom, when and for what?

Previous and Current Medical History
(*Basic dataset*)

Previous Medical History
Diagnoses
Current Conditions

Allergies
- Allergen(s)
- Reaction
- Details of exposure & time course
- Clinician assessment of causation

Medication Details (for each medicine)
- Drug
- Dose
- Form
- Route
- Frequency
- Directions/Administration Instructions
- Duration of therapy (start/stop/review date)

ADRs
- Reaction
- Causative agent
- Details of exposure and time course
- Clinician assessment of causation

Pathology Tests
- Test type
- Result
- Time of Test

Community Pharmacy Consultation
(*For counselling about long term conditions*)
- Current medication, and how it is being taken (including other OTC medicines and herbal medicines)
- Recent medication.
- GP details
- Recent visit(s) to GP
- Any recent referrals (including GP, AE, MIU visits), to whom, when and for what?
- Social care Issues (e.g. elderly care support being supplied)
- Compliance aids used
- Recent Referral
- New Referral
- Pregnancy status
- Breast-feeding status
- Ethnicity/Family History

Acute Hospital Admission

(*Information required when a patient is admitted to hospital acutely unwell*)

- Age
- Weight
- Current medication, and how it is being taken (including other OTC medicines and herbal medicines)
- Recent medication
- GP details
- Recent visit(s) to GP
- Any recent referrals (including GP, AE, MIU visits), to whom, when and for what?
- Allergies and sensitivities
- Concurrent conditions/Previous Medical History
- Recent Tests
- Social care Issues (e.g. elderly care support being supplied)
- Compliance aids used
- Devices/appliances used and patient understanding of them.
- Pregnant/Breastfeeding (women of childbearing age)
- Ethnicity/Family History
- Social History
- Smoking history
- Alcohol and other recreational drugs
- Contact details for community pharmacist
- Formulation issues (swallowing, other special requirements)
- Admitting Consultant
- Mental Capacity
- Advance Directives in place

During Hospital Episode

(*information to be recorded when changes are made during the patient's hospital episode*)

- Reason(s) for any changes
- Rationale for therapy where appropriate including any trials that may have been undertaken.
- Records of any drug which was started and stopped during an admission, but which may affect ongoing, long term care (this should also be included in discharge information).

Hospital Discharge

(*information to be recorded when the patient is discharged from hospital*)

- Any final counselling/education that is given on discharge and any follow up actions that have been recommended.
- Any adverse events that have occurred related to medicines administered during the hospital stay.
- Any medicine-specific follow up that will be required e.g. INR, digoxin test etc.
- Relevant information about where ongoing supply to come from (if there are specific supply issues) (and if appropriate who will administer).

- Any Care Management Plan (CMP) that should be undertaken
- Contact details for regular community pharmacist and GP
- Contact details for main hospital pharmacy contact
- DDA or other social care requirements for support e.g. delivery
- Expected date of discharge
- Discharge method (clinical advice or self-discharge)
- Type of discharge destination (e.g. home or residential home)
- Physical and mental assessment.

Medicines Reviews
(*details required in addition to the basic dataset and pharmacy consultation data if a medicine review is carried out*)
- Type of MUR (annual/intervention)
- MUR requested by (patient/pharmacist/other)
- Consent for MUR obtained (oral/written)
- Name(s) of any other persons present
- Date of Review
- Location of Review (if not in pharmacy)
- PCO permission for off-site review
- Action Plan (Issue/Recommendation/Responsible Professional)
- Does patient use the medicine as prescribed? (Yes/No)
- Does patient know why they are using the medicine? (Yes/No)
- Does patient need more information on the medicine? (Yes/No)
- Is the formulation appropriate? (Yes/No)
- how medicines are stored, handled and used
- physical barriers
- concordance
- device use for medicine administration and monitoring (pens, inhalers, spacers, blood glucose meters)
- advice given about device use & counselling given
- contact details for all relevant healthcare professionals

Specific Details for Emergency Supply at Patient's Request
(*additional data items for a pharmacy emergency supply*)
- Date Rx last issued
- Date of last repeat review
- Date of next repeat review
- Patient consent
- Has patient been referred from elsewhere?
- Diagnosis
- Problems/Notes
- Details of other emergency supplies
- Reason for any refusal of previous emergency supplies
- Cost of previous emergency supplies
- GP details
- Regular pharmacy

- Next of kin
- Prescribing history
- Details of onward referral

Shared Care
(*additional data items if a medicine is prescribed on a shared care arrangement*)
- Identity of the medicines – what is it, what does it do, how is it being used
- Who is responsible (inc their role) for:
  - Initiation
  - Monitoring
  - Ongoing supply (including prescribing/prescription source)
  - Review
  - Decision to stop
  - Contact details for all of above
  - Information given to the patient/carer
  - Main contact for any problems or questions
- Copy of or links to shared care agreement or protocol
- Where can information about the 'unusual' medicine be found (i.e. reference source)
- Cross link with other information already identified in previous cases – remember to include e.g. coils, herbal preps etc.
- High risk medicines – highlight

Emergency Hospital Admission: Patient Unconscious
(*information required if a patient is admitted to hospital unconscious*)
- Patient ID
- Emergency medical treatment/Pre hospital care
- Current medication, and how it is being taken (including OTC medicines and herbal medicines)
- Recent medication and reasons for stopping.
- Any recent referrals (including GP, AE, MIU visits), to whom, when and for what?
- Allergies and sensitivities
- ADRs
- Concurrent conditions/Previous Medical History
- Recent Tests
- Admitting consultant
- Mental capacity
- Any advance directives in place

Management of Long Term Conditions
(*additional information required for management of patients with long term conditions*)
- Clinical Management Plan
- Review Dates required for all long term conditions
- Expiry/Storage of Medicines
- Compliance Information
- Other Healthcare Professionals involved in the patient's care
- Repeat dispensing of when required (PRN) medicines

Homecare Supply
(*additional information required for management of patients receiving homecare supplies*)
• Nominated pharmacy
• Details of what other health professionals need to know from the pharmacy
• Special Administration Instructions
• Details of the healthcare professional administering the drug (name, organization, contact number etc.)
• Monitoring requirements
• Communications Notes (e.g. DNA)
• Details of related MURs
• Details of homecare company
• Details of procurement hub involved in purchase of the homecare package

Appliances
(*additional information required for patients with appliances or devices*)
• Type of Device/Appliance
• How often should it be used/changed?
• For how long is it required? (temporary (e.g. reversible stoma)/permanent)
• Dm+d code(s)
• Specific details of where the device can be obtained (inc phone ordering or helpline)
• Details on likely supply delays
• Is there a centralised (PCT wide) supply system?
• When and how often should treatment progress be monitored?

Appliance/Device Specific Information

Stoma Care

A unique identifier is needed as codes differ between primary and secondary care, to enable tariff manipulation.
• What set of products are needed for the patient? As well as bags, all accessories should be listed.

Diabetes Care

• Which pump/device is being used?
• What needles are required?
• What blood glucose test machine and strips are required?
• Can blood glucose meter download data directly into computerised records?
• Has a sharps bin been supplied and patient briefed on sharps disposal?
• For children/young people, is insulin being administered at school?

Catheters

A unique identifier is needed as codes differ between primary and secondary care, to enable tariff manipulation.
• Male/Female
• Urethral/Suprapubic catheter
• Gauge
• Latex allergy (although latex less often used)
• Actual instructions for changing catheter (may differ from manufacturer's recommendation)

Nebulisers

• How to maintain equipment
• Instructions on when to treat exacerbations (antibiotics/steroids/changes of dose of inhaled medication)

Dressings

• Size of dressing
• Shape of dressing
• Type of dressing
• Reason for use
• How often the dressing should be changed
• Who is changing the dressing?
• Instructions for dealing with infection
• Order of application if more than one dressing is used concomitantly

First Aid
(*information required to record first aid incidents in the pharmacy*)
• The background to the incident
• Treatment given to patient
• Advice/information given to patient
• Details of suspected underlying disease
• Referral made

Medicines Administration
(*information required to enable pharmacist support for special methods of medicine administration*)
• Compliance aid?
• Enteral tubes? (PEG tube, NG tube etc.)
• Lines? (Hickman line etc.)
• Syringe driver – details of device and delivery rate
• Liquid required

- SF formulation required
- Nebulizer required
- Compliance issues
- DDA assessment performed
- Are special adminisitration requirements long or short-term?
- Date of last medication review
- Date of next medication review

Patient Group Directions
(*additional information required for management of patients receiving medicines supplied on patient group directions*)
- PGD instructions and conditions
- Prescribing history
- Previous PGD supplies
- Previous refusal to supply on PGD and reasons
- Patient identifier – to enable patient anonymity
- Pharmacist's credentials & authorisation
- Diagnostic tests performed
- Results of diagnostic tests performed

Public Health and Disease Screening
(*information required to enable pharmacy provision of public health services*)
- Does subject consent to screening service
- Age
- Weight
- Height
- BMI
- Current medication, and how it is being taken (including other OTC medicines and herbal medicines)
- Recent medication
- Any recent referrals (including GP, AE, MIU visits), to whom, when and for what?
- Allergies and sensitivities
- Concurrent conditions/Previous Medical History
- Recent Tests
- Pregnant/Breastfeeding (women of childbearing age)
- Ethnicity/Family History
- Social History
- Smoking history
- Alcohol and other recreational drugs
- Record of advice given to subject
- Does subject consent to findings being sent to GP
- Does subject reject advice given

Clinic
(*additional information required for pharmacists providing clinic services*)
Information required is as for *Public Health & Disease Screening* (above) and also:

- Patient issues (e.g. witness protection, child protection)
- Does patient consent to the clinic appointment?
- Relevant NPSA alerts

Specific clinic requirements, for example:

- Smoking
  - FEV1
  - CO
- Diabetic
  - HBA1C
  - Blood sugar series
- Warfarin
  - INR etc.

Home Visits

(*additional information required to support home visits by pharmacists*)

- Basic Information and also:
- Repeat prescription/dispensing frequency
- Date of next repeat supply
- Date of next review
- Name of official carer
- Name of informal carer(s)
- Information about carer ability

Referrals

(*information to support recording of referral details by pharmacists*)

Basic information and also:

- Patient's consent to the transfer of information
- Reason for referral
- Details of referring professional & qualifications
- Relevant recommendations
- Request for acknowledgement of referral (where necessary)

This basic framework for the Standard Pharmaceutical Care Record was developed and presented by the Royal Pharmaceutical Society at a stakeholder engagement event in April 2010. http://www.rpharms.com/archive-events/sciconf100426.pdf

Appendix C: Classification Framework for Pharmacy Interventions

The Royal Pharmaceutical Society of Great Britain has previously issued guidance on the recording of interventions giving advice on when to record interventions, where to record interventions and how long to retain intervention records for. However, while the guidance gives outline advice on what information to record, this is not covered in detail.

Use of a standard classification would ensure that numbers and types of interventions are easily comparable and that these can be used to formulate statistical data on service use and efficacy.

The Welsh Chief Pharmacists' Guidelines on the Provision of Pharmaceutical Care[1] stated that: "*as a result of a pharmacy review each patient will receive the* **right** *dose of medicine, at the* **right** *time, with the* **right** *dose schedule, the* **right** *route of administration and for the* **right** *duration*".

The following proposed classification of pharmacy interventions is based on these requirements and also relevant pharmacy literature.

Proposed Standard Classification for Pharmacy Interventions

1. Right Medicine Interventions
   * 1.1 Unnecessary Medicine
   * 1.2 Duplication of Medicine
   * 1.3 Incorrect Medicine (Transcription Error)
   * 1.4 Medicine Reconciliation Query (query with patient)
   * 1.5 Inappropriate Medicine for Indication/Patient Condition
   * 1.6 Inappropriate Medicine for patient allergies/sensitivities
   * 1.7 Inappropriate Medicine because of absolute contraindications
   * 1.9 Unlicensed Use
   * 1.10 Need for additional medicine (adjuvant therapy)

2. Right Dose Interventions
   * 2.1 Dose too high
   * 2.2 Dose too low
   * 2.3 Inappropriate Dose for Indication/Patient Condition
   * 2.4 Unlicensed Dose

3. Right Frequency/Dose Schedule Interventions
   * 3.1 Dose Frequency Incorrect
   * 3.2 Inappropriate Dose Frequency for Indication/Patient Condition

4. Right Duration of Treatment Interventions
   (for medicines where duration of treatment is significant)
   * 4.1 Duration of Treatment not specified
   * 4.2 Review period not specified
   * 4.3 Inappropriate Continuation of Treatment Period
   * 4.4 Inappropriate Discontinuation of Treatment Period
   * 4.5 Compliance/Concordance Issues

5. Right Therapy Intervention
   * 5.1 Adverse Drug Reaction (ADR)
   * 5.2 Clinically Significant Drug Interaction
   * 5.3 Therapeutic Drug Monitoring (TDM) Query

---

[1] Welsh Chief Pharmacists guidelines on the provision of pharmaceutical care, vol 2; 2009

6. Right Administration Interventions
   - 6.1 Inappropriate Route of Administration for Indication/Patient Condition
   - 6.2 Inappropriate Route of Administration for Pharmaceutical Form of Medicine
   - 6.3 Route of Administration not specified
   - 6.4 Choice of Routes of Administration required but not specified
   - 6.5 Incorrect Method of Medicine Administration
   - 6.6 Inappropriate Method of Medicine Administration for the patient's needs

7. Right Prescription Interventions
   - 7.1 Prescription not legal
   - 7.2 Prescription is for a non-formulary product

Appendix D: Pharmacy IT Select Bibliography

IT Basics for Pharmacists
Fisher R. Information technology for pharmacists. Pharmaceutical Press: London; 2006

Pharmacy Informatics
Fox BI, Thrower MR, Felkey BG. Building core competencies in pharmacy informatics. American Pharmacists Association: Washington DC; 2010
Dumitru D, Gumpper K. The pharmacy informatics primer. ASHP Publications: Bethesda; 2009
Anderson PO, McGuinness SM, Bourne PE. Pharmacy informatics. CRC Press: Boca Raton; 2010

Clinical Decision Support
Osheroff J. Improving outcomes with clinical decision support: an implemneter's guide. Healthcare Information & Management Systems Society: Chicago; 2012

Electronic Prescribing
Goundrey-Smith SJ. Principles of electronic prescribing. Springer: London; 2008

Electronic Transfer of Prescriptions (E-Prescribing – US Context)
Fincham JE. E-prescribing: the electronic transformation of medicine. Jones & Bartlett: Sudbury; 2009.
Van Ornum M. Electronic prescribing: a safety and implementation guide. Jones & Bartlett: Sudbury; 2009.

Index

A
ADEs. *See* Adverse drug events (ADEs)
Adverse drug events (ADEs), 61, 62, 69
Adverse drug reactions, 133
Asset tracking, 191
Automated systems, 187
Automated unit-dose drug distribution
    system, 64–65

B
Barcode identification, 177, 181
Barcode medicines administration (BCMA)
  anaesthetics, cardiac surgery cases, 68
  cabinets, 108
  cardiac surgery cases, 188
  medication errors and patient safety, 68
  work-around, 188
Barcodes, 67–69
Barcodes and logistics
  description, 175–176
  e-commerce, pharmacy, 185–186
  electronic medicines administration
    BCMA, 187, 188
    drug trolley, 188
    potential barriers, 189
    RFID, 189
  intraoperability, 185
  issues, pharmacy and medicines
    management, 175
  optical technology
    2D bar codes, 178–179
    GS1 barcode, 178
    product tracking, 179
    scanners, 178
  patient safety, 182–184

  pharmaceutical distribution processes
    DTP supply, 176
    EAN code, 177
    PIP code, 177
    stock control, 176
    traditional distribution systems, 177
    unlicensed medicines, 176
  pharmacy workflow tracking, 189–191
  reduction, dispensing errors, 186–187
  RFID, 179
  security, supply chain, 184
  supply chain harmonisation
    cross-industry working group, 180–181
    EHR, 180
    NDC, 179
    standard coding system, 180
  symbology harmonisation
    international coding standard, 181
    seamless pharmaceutical supply
     chain, 182
    stakeholders, 182
  tracking, supply chain efficiency, 184–185
  use, 191
Batch numbers, 178
BCMA. *See* Barcode medicines
    administration (BCMA)
Blister pack, 198
Blood glucose readings, 203

C
Cancer outcomes and services dataset
    (COSD), 12
CAP. *See* Common assurance process (CAP)
Central intravenous additives (CIVAS), 157
Chronic diseases, 202, 203

CIVAS. *See* Central intravenous
     additives (CIVAS)
Clinical Knowledge Summaries (CKS), 16
Coding
     allergies, 11
     benefits, patient care, 14
     care management, 14
     COSD, 12
     dm + d structure, 14
     DRGs, 12
     GP systems, 124–126
     health level 7 (HL7), 13
     health statistics, 11
     ICD-CM, 12
     medicine item, 15
     methodologies, 11
     NHS, 13
     pharmacy domains, 11
     read codes, 12
     SNOMED, 13
     UK Prescription Pricing Authority, 13–14
Commissioning for Quality and Innovation
     (CQUIN), 100
Common assurance process (CAP), 25, 164
Complex administration instructions, 79
Computerized physician order entry
     (CPOE), 60, 61, 69
Continuing professional development
     (CPD), 126, 213
Contraindications, 72
COSD. *See* Cancer outcomes and services
     dataset (COSD)
CPD. *See* Continuing professional
     development (CPD)
CPOE. *See* Computerized physician order
     entry (CPOE)
CQUIN. *See* Commissioning for Quality
     and Innovation (CQUIN)

D
Data Migration Improvement Project
     (DMIP), 134
Decision support (DS), 71–76, 133
Decision support systems (DSS)
     adverse reactions, 129
     care pathway management, 131
     contra-indications, 129
     diagnosis, 131
     drug database, 130
     duplicate therapy, 129
     EPS, 130
     functions, GPs, 129
     generic substitution, 129

     medicine cost information, 129
     pharmacy system, 129
     repeat prescriptions, 130
     transfer, care date, 131
Diagnosis related groups (DRGs)
     codes, 10
     ICD-CM, 12
     medicine cost data, 12
     reimbursement algorithm, 12
Digital television, 202, 203
Direct to purchaser (DTP), 176
Dispensing errors, 102–103
Dispensing process efficiency, 103
DMIP. *See* Data Migration Improvement
     Project (DMIP)
DRGs. *See* Diagnosis related groups (DRGs)
Drug charts, 63
Drug interactions, 72
DS. *See* Decision support (DS)
DSS. *See* Decision support systems (DSS)
DTP. *See* Direct to purchaser (DTP)

E
EAN code. *See* European Article Number
     (EAN) code
E-commerce, 185–186
EDI. *See* Electronic data interchange (EDI)
EHR. *See* Electronic health records (EHR)
Electronic data interchange (EDI), 186
Electronic dissemination, prescriptions, 86–87
Electronic drug databases
     automated systems, 18
     hospital EP systems, 19
     ISO 9001, 20
     MicroMedex, 18
     pharmacy application, 19–20
Electronic drug trolley, 188
Electronic health records (EHR)
     allergies, 34
     benefits
          decision support tools, 45
          PIM, 46
          polypharmacy, 46
          record security, 45
          transformative technology, 47
     design and use
          archiving and destruction, records, 41
          business continuity, 40
          creation, EPRs, 35–36
          definition, 34
          EPR, 39
          liability, record use, 37–38
          pharmacy professionals, 36–37

sharing, data, 39–40
subject access, 38–39
system, EPRs, 34–35
use of data, 40
healthcare professionals, 27
hospital pharmacy systems, 171
legal and professional framework
    confidentiality, 29
    consent, 30
    liability, 30
medical history, 34
and NHS IT systems, 185
PAS, 154
patient demographic data, 154
pharmacy claims, 166
product information, 184
Electronic information sources
CKS, 16
drug information, 15
drug interactions/drugs in pregnancy, 16
EMBASE, 16
EMC, 18
EPAD, 17
medical information, 16, 17
PDR and MIMS, 16
pharmaceutical industry and regulatory
    agencies, 16–17
PIL, 17
Electronic medicine administration, 82
Electronic medicines management, primary
    care
CPD, 122
data quality, 126
development, systems
    dispensing, medicines, 121–122
    medical and pharmacy practice, 122
    VA, 123
ETP, 135–147
GPs
    clinical coding, 124–126
    consultation workflow, 131
    data migration, 134
    document management, 132–133
    DSS, 129–131
    GP2GP transfer, 133
    pathology tests, 131–132
    patients and registration, 127
    problem and episode recording,
        127–128
    recording, allergies, 128–129
    record keeping, 126
    reimbursement claim, 131
    safety and usability, 134–135
health economies, 121

medication-related patient
    information, 148
prescribing software
    activity analysis, 148
    benchmarking, 148
    budget management, 148
    commissioning information
        systems, 148
    invoice validation, 148
    KP, 147
    PCT, 147
    QMAS, 147
    QoF, 147
Electronic patient records (EPR)
    applications, pharmacists
        allergy, 49
        medicines reconciliation, 50
        MUR, 50
    benefits EHRs, 45–47
    clinical pathways and content, 47–48
    creation, 35–36
    design and use, EHR (see Electronic
        health records (EHR))
    development, 28–29
    EHR system, 28
    healthcare professionals, 27
    IG and data sharing (see Information
        governance (IG))
    initiatives, 41–45
    legal and professional framework, EHR,
        29–30
    PCR (see Pharmaceutical care record)
    pharmaceutical care, 48–49
    PMR system, 27
    quality, care, 27
    systems used, 34–35
Electronic prescribing (EP) system
    benefits, 60–61
    care benefits, 88–89
    clinical system intraoperability, 85–86
    description, 59
    discharge process efficiency, 82–83
    hospital business processes, 86–87
    NHS, 60
    paediatrics
        barcodes, 67–69
        complex dosing schedules, 66
        electronic decision support tools, 71–76
        evaluating risk reduction, 76–78
        increases, medication errors, 69–70
        POE and NOE, 67
    paper and consumables, 85
    reduction, medication error
        rates (see Medication error rates)

Electronic prescribing (EP) system (*cont.*)
  seamless pharmaceutical supply chain,
    83–84
  security, 88
  sociopolitical developments, 59
  sociotechnical systems, 89–90
  workflow management (*see* Workflow
    management)
Electronic prescription service (EPS), 153
Electronic transfer of prescriptions (ETP)
  accuracy checking, 144
  adoption
    pharmacy roles, 147
    secondary care, 146
  barcode, 136
  benefits
    communication channel, 137
    community pharmacy, 137
    decision support functions, 137
    dose syntax model, 136
    information governance, 136–137
    repeat dispensing, 137
    workflow design, 136
  business continuity, 146
  cancellation, electronic prescriptions, 145
  controlled drugs, 136
  data structure and product selection
    mapping, 146
    pharmacy systems, 146
    prescribing token, 146
  dispense notification, 144
  electronic repeat dispensing, 145–146
  EP, 135
  functionality issues
    access management, 138
    access, systems, 138
    dispense notification, 139
    dispensing tokens, 141
    e-commerce, 139
    electronic prescription, 141–142
    electronic repeat dispensing, 139
    electronic signatures, 139
    emergency supply, 142
    EPS Release 1 and 2, 142
    national spine, 142
    patients identification, 141–142
    PCT, 138
    pharmacy nomination, 139–140
    prescription retrieval, 140–141
    prescription tokens, 140
    Registration Authority, 138
    reimbursement endorsement
     messages, 139
    system requirements, 138

labelling
  configuration options, 144
  dose syntax, 144
  electronic, 144
  legal entity, 136
  national spine, 136
  nominated pharmacy, 136
  personal administration, 136
  primary care team, 121
  professional checking
    pharmacy systems, 143
    prescription messages, 143
  Regenstrief Rx Hub, 135
  reimbursement endorsement messages, 145
  stock items, 144
  substitution, 143
  supplementary clinical information,
    142–143
Electronic ward cabinets
  benefits, 109–110
  description, 106
  implementation issues, 110–112
  medicines management, 109
  number, issues, 108–109
  pharmacy stock control, 108
Emergency Care Summary (ECS),
    Scotland, 123
E-ordering, 185
EP. *See* Electronic prescribing (EP)
EPAD. *See* European Public Assessment
    Document (EPAD)
EPR. *See* Electronic patient records (EPR)
EPS. *See* Electronic prescription service (EPS)
EP system. *See* Electronic prescribing (EP)
    system
ETP. *See* Electronic transfer of prescriptions
    (ETP)
European Article Number (EAN) code, 97,
    178, 180, 181
European Public Assessment Document
    (EPAD), 17
Expiry dates, 109, 178

G
General medical practice systems (GPs)
  clinical coding
    classification, 124
    code substitution process, 126
    primary care, 124
    semantic scope, 125, 126
    SNOMED, 124
    UK National Health Service, 124
  data quality, 126

functionality
  data migration, 134
  document management, 132–133
  DSS, 129–131
  and episode recording, 127–128
  GP2GP transfer, 133
  identification, patients and
      registration, 127
  items, service, 131
  pathology tests, 131–132
  recording, allergies, 128–129
  record keeping, 126
safety and usability
  audit trails, 135
  decision support, 134
  electronic prescribing, 134
  prescribing workflow, 135
  repeat prescribing, 135
  triadic consultation, 135
  UAR, 135
GPs. See General medical practice
      systems (GPs)
GPSoC. See GP Systems of Choice (GPSoC)
GP Systems of Choice (GPSoC), 122

H
Healthcare management organizations
      (HMOs)
  dynamics, working, 137
  integrated care, 41
  KP, 28
  long term conditions, 41
  payor, 145
  Regenstrief medication hub, 166
  regional systems, 28
  VA and KP, 41
HIS. See Hospital information system (HIS)
HMOs. See Healthcare management
      organizations (HMOs)
Homecare company, 206–207
Hospital information system (HIS)
  PAS, 10
  pharmacy/stock control functionality, 168
Human error, 183

I
ICD. See International classification of
      diseases (ICD)
IDS. See Immediate discharge summaries
      (IDS)
IG. See Information governance (IG)
Immediate discharge summaries (IDS), 82

Individual Health Record (IHR), Wales, 123
Information governance (IG)
  data sharing
      description, 31
      patient information, 31
      PCTs, 32
  requirements, 88
  UK health records standards initiatives
      developing standards, recommendation,
        33–34
      primary care, 32–33
      RCP, 33
      SRPG, 32
International classification of diseases (ICD)
  CM codes, 12
  ICD 10, 11–12
Intraoperability
  clinical system, 85–86
  coding systems, 10
  HIS, 10
  HMOs and stakeholders, 11
  PAS, 9

K
Kaiser Permanente (KP), 28, 147

L
Legitimate relationship (LR)
  RBAC, 37
  types
      clinician self claimed, 44
      patient self referral, 44
LR. See Legitimate relationship (LR)

M
MAR. See Medicines administration record
      (MAR)
Medical wards, 109
Medication error rates
  ADEs, 62
  complexity level, 65
  controlled and intravenous drugs, 64
  CPOE, 61
  discharge prescribing error, 63
  drug chart, 62, 63
  financial cost, 61
  implementation period, 61–62
  "kardex" systems, 64
  pharmacy intervention scheme, 63
  quantitative studies, 66
Medicine administration errors, 95, 110

Medicines administration. *See* Electronic
    prescribing (EP)
Medicines administration record
    (MAR), 156
Medicines use review (MUR),
    50, 157
Medicine-taking behaviours, 201
Methadone dispensing, 114
Mobile phone, 202, 203, 205
MUR. *See* Medicines use review (MUR)

N
National Drug Code (NDC), 179
National Health Service (NHS), 59, 84
NDC. *See* National Drug
    Code (NDC)
New Medicines Service (NMS), 170
NHS. *See* National Health Service (NHS)
NMS. *See* New Medicines Service (NMS)
NOE. *See* Nurse order entry (NOE)
Nurse order entry (NOE), 67

O
Oncology systems, 196
Optical light-beam technology, 96

P
Paediatrics, medication error rates
    barcodes, 67–69
    description, 66
    electronic decision support tools
        action plans, 76
        applications and benefits, 73–75
        chronic diseases, 76
        clinical decision, 71
        contraindications, 72
        drug database, 72
        DS applications, 73
        formulary medicines, non-formulary
            medicines, 73
        monitoring, 71
        patient record, 72
        warning fatigue, 72
    EP systems
        ADEs, 69, 70
        CPOE implementation, 69
        human-machine interface, 69
        prescribing error, 70
    POE and NOE, 67
    risk reduction, evaluation, 76–78

Paper and consumables, 85
PAS. *See* Patient administration system (PAS)
Pathology Messaging Implementation
    Project (PMIP)
    units, measurement, 132
    web-based technology, 132
Pathology systems, 161, 194
Pathology test, 86, 87
Patient administration system (PAS)
    demographic data, 194
    EHR, 28
    enterprise-based, 28
    HIS, 10
    secondary care, 9
Patient group direction (PGD), 55
Patient information leaflet (PIL), 17
Patient medication record
    (PMR) systems
    allergy and interactions, 49
    community pharmacy, 34
    hospitals and community, 27
    retail pharmacy, 162
    UK community, 151
Patient safety
    audit commission's spoonful of sugar
        report, 182
    EHR, 184
    human error, 183
    medication error rates, 183
    medication errors, 183
    SOPs, 183
Patients own drugs (PODs), 159
PCTs. *See* Primary care trusts (PCTs)
PDOs. *See* Pre-defined orders (PDOs)
Peristaltic pumps, 115
PGD. *See* Patient group direction (PGD)
Pharmaceutical care record
    ADRs/allergies, 51
    appliances, 54–55
    description, 50
    EHR, 50
    homecare supply, 54
    home visits, 55
    long term condition management, 53
    medicines reconciliation, 52–53
    medicines reviews, 51–52
    PGD supply (*see* Patient group direction
        (PGD))
    pharmacist, 51
    public health and screening, 55
    shared care, 53
    social information, 51
Pharmaceutical industry, 175, 178, 184

Pharmacy automation
    benefits, electronic ward cabinets, 110
    benefits of robots
        dispensing process efficiency, 103–104
        dispensing systems, 105
        reduction, dispensing errors, 102–103
        use of space, pharmacy, 104
    dispensary technology, 96
    drivers for use, 100, 102
    electronic ward cabinets, 106–109
    evaluation, benefits, 105–107
    implementation issues, electronic ward
        cabinets, 110, 112
    medicine administration errors, 95
    methadone dispensing, 96
    remote dispensing systems, 112–113
    robot design and operation, 97–98
    robots and remote dispensing, 95
    specialist dispensing systems
        benefits, 115
        consultation areas, 117
        interpersonal factors, 115
        medicines management, 116
        methadone dispensing, 114
        methameasure, 115, 116
        NHS reforms, 114
        peristaltic pumps, 115
        supervised consumption, 114
    UK
        ARX ROWA speedcase device, 98
        business case, 99
        dispensary robot, 100, 101
        hospital pharmacy robot
            implementations, 99, 100
        off-site centralized medicine supply, 99
Pharmacy distribution centre, 99
Pharmacy, information technology (IT)
    applications, clinical, 193–194
    benefits, 193
    clinical homecare, 206–207
    clinical pharmacy, 21–22
    clinical safety, 23–24
    coding, medicines concepts, 11–14
    consumerism, 2
    demographic data, 194
    description, 1
    development, clinical pharmacy, 6–7
    device integration, 196–197
    education and training
        British Computer Society, 215
        competencies cover, 214
        CPD, 213
        hardware and software, 213

    and orientation, healthcare, 212
    profession, 214
    electronic drug databases, 18–20
    empowered patient, 2
    EP, 195
    healthcare, 7–9
    health strategy, 211
    inertia, professional engagement,
        211–212
    interface and integration, 194
    internet, 1
    intraoperability, 9–11
    medicine item codes, 15
    medicines, 20–21
    medicines information, 2
    medicines management, 193
    methodology and evaluation, 207–208
    modes of action, 1
    NHS, 2
    oncology systems, 196
    pharmaceutical industry, 1
    pharmacists, 1
    pharmacopoeias and compendia, 1
    pharmacy vs. pharmaceutical industry,
        22–23
    professional standards, 208–210
    profession, pharmacy, 4–6
    public health and budgets, 2
    purpose and scope
        adoption and use, technology, 3
        EHR and EP, 3
        eTP and prescribing management
            systems, 3
        GP systems, 3
        pharmacy managers, 2
        pharmacy profession, 4
    service development, 211
    smart packaging (see Smart packaging)
    smart pumps, 195–196
    sociotechnical innovation, 24–25
    support tools, 194
    systems-based approach, 210
    telecare (see Telecare)
Pharmacy management systems
    architecture
        community, 155
        electronic signature, 155
        finance, 154
        hospital pharmacy, 154
        monitored dose, 154
        pathology, 154
        pharmacy robot, 154
    automation, 171

Pharmacy management systems (*cont.*)
  benefits
    allergies, 165
    data fragmentation issues, 166
    decision support, 165
    departmental workflow, 164
    HMOs, 164
    medication errors, 165
    pathology test result, 166
    Regenstrief medication hub, 166
  clinical and medicines information,
    162–163
  community functions
    diagnostic screening, 157
    dispensing cycles, 156
    drug interactions, 156
    drug tariff, 156
    endorsement support, 155
    labelling, 155
    MAR, 156
    MUR, 157
    PAS, 156
    patient medication record, 155
    prescribing/dispensing decision
      support, 155
    product pricing, 155
    professional activity, 155
    repeat dispensing, 156
    stock control and ordering, 155
  definition, 151
  departmental IT applications
    pharmacokinetics, 167
    therapeutic drug monitoring, 167
    TPN, 167–168
  EP functions, 168
  fridge temperature monitoring software,
    169–170
  functions
    business continuity, 164
    CAP, 164
    client–server architecture, 163
    database structure, 163
    drug data updates, 163
  history and development
    adoption, 152
    hospital mainframe, 152
    order entry, 151
    patient demographic information, 152
    pharmacokinetic calculations, 151
    ward stock lists, 151
  hospital functions
    chemotherapy, 157
    CIVAS, 157
    clinical homecare, 157
    commissioning processes, 158
    electronic prescribing, 158
    pathology systems, 158
    patient medication record, 157
    pharmacy systems, 158
    requirements, 157
    stock control database, 158
    TPN, 157
  integrated community, 170
  interfaces, 160–161
  reporting, 161–162
  requirements and use
    drug-related problems, 153
    EPS, 153
    PMR, 153
    stock control, 152
  Sonar informatics, 170
  stock control methodologies, 158–160
Pharmacy robot
  benefits, 102–106
  design and operation, 97–98
Pharmacy robots, 161
Physician order entry (POE), 67
PIL. *See* Patient information leaflet (PIL)
PMIP. *See* Pathology Messaging
    Implementation Project (PMIP)
PMR. *See* Patient medication record (PMR)
PODs. *See* Patients own drugs (PODs)
POE. *See* Physician order entry (POE)
Pre-defined orders (PDOs), 80
Primary care trusts (PCTs)
  IG agenda, 32
  networked GP systems, 147
  pharmacists, 55
Product security, 184
Product tracking, 184, 185

Q
QIPP. *See* Quality, Innovation, Productivity
    and Prevention
QMAS. *See* Quality management and analysis
    system (QMAS)
QoF. *See* Quality and outcomes framework
    (QoF)
Quality and outcomes framework
    (QoF), 147
Quality, care benefits, 88–89
Quality, Innovation, Productivity
    and Prevention (QIPP), 100
Quality management and analysis system
    (QMAS), 147

R

Radio frequency product identification
(RFID), 179, 191
RBAC. *See* Role based access (RBAC)
RCP. *See* Royal College of Physicians
(RCP)
Recording
allergies
data transfer process, 129
decision support system, 128–129
GP2GP, 129
medication (*see* Decision support
systems (DSS))
problem and episode
diagnoses, 127
FNO, 128
life events, 127
management, 128
symptoms, 127
Remote dispensing systems, 95, 112–113
Reporting
business and service management, 161
departmental activity reports, 162
most frequently used item report, 162
non-compliant patient reports, 162
outpatient prescribing, 162
owed products report, 162
patient histories, 162
prescription throughput reports, 162
reimbursement claim estimates, 162
residual stock reports, 162
service provision targets, 162
Role based access (RBAC), 37
Royal College of Physicians (RCP), 33

S

SCR. *See* Summary care record (SCR)
Seamless pharmaceutical supply chain,
83–84, 175, 182
Sensitivity checking, 71–72
Shared Record Professional Guidance (SRPG)
project, 32, 123
Smartcard, 88
Smart pack, 197–201
Smart packaging
blister packs, 200
data, 198
device manufacturer, 199
electronic devices, 198–199
medicines, 197–198
monitoring technologies, 201
non-adherence, 197

patients, 201
technical standards, 199
SmPC. *See* Summary of product
characteristics (SmPC)
SNOMED. *See* Systematised nomenclature
of medicine (SNOMED)
SOPs. *See* Standard operating procedures
(SOPs)
Standard operating procedures (SOPs), 183
Stock control, 96, 108, 114
Stock control methodologies, hospitals
28 day (one stop) dispensing, 160
devices, 158
discharge process, 160
dispensing, UK, 159
electronic ward cabinets, 158
medicine chart, 159
notional cost, 159
pharmacy automation, 158
pharmacy robots, 158
PODs, 159
unit dose activity, 158
Summary care record (SCR)
clinician self claimed LR, 44
descrption, 30
elements of information, 42
medicines reconciliation, 52
patient self referral LR, 44
in pharmacy settings, 42
unscheduled care, 42
Summary of product characteristics (SmPC)
and PIL, 17
UK authorizations, 17
Surgical wards, 109
Swiss cheese effect, 183
Syringe driver, 195
Systematised nomenclature of medicine
(SNOMED)
classifications of tumour, 13
CT, 13
SNOMED III, 13

T

Telecare
appropriate technology, 202
barriers, 205–206
blood glucose results, 205
chronic diseases, 202, 203
development programme, 204
digital television, 203
healthcare, 202
hypertension, 204

Telecare (*cont.*)
    mobile phone, 203
    patient care processes, 201
    personalized medicine, 204
    telemedicine, 205
Telemedicine, 204–205
Therapeutic revolution, 68
Total parenteral nutrition (TPN),
    167–168
TPN. *See* Total parenteral nutrition
    (TPN)

U
UAR. *See* User action
    recording (UAR)
UK Royal Pharmaceutical Society, 140
Unit-dose dispensing, 95, 97–98
User action recording (UAR), 135

V
VA. *See* Veterans Administration (VA)
Veterans Administration (VA), 123

W
Workflow management
    confirmation boxes, 80
    continuous infusions, 82
    electronic medicine administration, 82
    ethical requirements and legal
        requirements, 78
    layout design, 81
    legible and complete prescription, 78
    medicines administration, 80
    PDOs, 80
    screen prompts, 79
    secondary care, 79
    user code, 81

9781447158370